Contents

Foreword by Alex Jack   5

1. Basics and Benefits of Macrobiotics   7
2. Yin and Yang in Social Organization   17
3. The Beauty of Rice Fields   20
4. A Unifying Cosmology   22
5. Diet and Behavior   24
6. Conversations with T. Colin Campbell   30
7. Teaching Macrobiotics in Southern California   36
8. Relativity   41
9. Reflections on the Philosopher's Stone   43
10. Seminars in Belgium and France   49
11. Planetary Medicine   56
12. Toward Planetary Family   58
13. Preventing Crime through Diet   62
14. New Reasons to be Dairy-free   66
15. Good Food and Gardening at Graterford   71
16. Macrobiotics in the Pacific Rim   74
17. Maintaining Optimal Weight   79
18. Adventures in Natural Farming   81
19. Freedom for Health   85
20. Health and Spiritual Development   87
21. Yuki Nabé (Snow Nabé)   91

Resources   92
Recommended Reading   93
About the Author   94
Index   95

Foreword

Over the last generation, macrobiotics has grown from a small circle of friends into a movement for planetary change. From Boston to Moscow, from Tokyo to Ridayh, from Singapore to Accra, macrobiotic teachers, cooks, and educational centers are guiding people to a healthier, more peaceful way of life and establishing new values and priorities for the coming century.

Hotels, schools, hospitals, and clinics are now actively seeking macrobiotic products and services to offer to their staff and the general public. In Boston recently, a large medical research conference sponsored by Harvard University and the World Health Organization featured a macrobiotic banquet for several hundred leading scientists from around the world.

Edward Esko, the author of this book, has been among the most active macrobiotic teachers over the last twenty years, lecturing and counseling in Europe, Asia, Latin America, and throughout North America and writing and editing numerous books and articles. Building on the teachings of George Ohsawa and Michio Kushi, he has applied yin and yang—the simple principles of balance and harmony—to helping to solve the environmental crisis, the plague of crime and violence in our communities, and other modern social ills.

Basics and Benefits of Macrobiotics recounts the author's most recent adventures, discoveries, and travels. Like a latter-day knight of the Round Table, we see him sallying forth through the nutritional landscape of present-day Europe, upholding the virtues of white sea salt against an array of detractors. Like a modern samurai swordsman, we see him plunging into the thicket of transmutation, conceiving of new ways to produce tungsten, steel, and other precious metals and defuse the approaching energy crisis between East and West. From Charlie Chaplin to Colin Campbell, he invokes prophets of balance and moderation who have foreseen the limits of modern civilization.

On his journeys, Edward continually offers practical advice to individuals and families. In these pages, we see him showing people how to prevent hyperactivity in children, reverse schizophrenia, overcome hypogycemia, and relieve a kidney stone. In macrobiotics, the personal and planetary are intertwined. When one person is nourished, the whole planet benefits. When the planet is healed, each person is cleansed and refreshed.

The essays in this book are part of the most exciting adventure in the world today—macrobiotics, the great life—to preserve our planet and ensure humanity's continued biological and spiritual evolution. Please digest its contents well, begin to implement principles of natural order in your own life, and join in the endless quest for universal health and peace.

> Alex Jack
> April 23, 1995
> Becket, Massachusetts

1.
Basics and Benefits of Macrobiotics

One of the most basic principles of macrobiotics is to eat an ecological, environmentally-based diet. That means to rely primarily on foods native to the climate and environment in which we live. Until the modern age, people were more or less dependent on the products of their regional agriculture. Foods that grew in their area formed the basis of their daily diet. It was not until modern technology that it became possible for people to base their diets on foods from regions with far different climates.

Today, it is common for people to consume bananas from South America, sugar from the Caribbean, pineapples from the South Pacific, or kiwi from New Zealand. However, our health depends on our ability to adapt to the changes in our environment. When we eat foods from a climate that is very different from ours, we lose that adaptability. As society moved away from its traditional, ecologically-based diet, there has been a corresponding rise in chronic illness. Therefore, for optimal health, we need to return to a way of eating based on foods produced in our local environment, or at least on foods grown in a climate that is similar to ours.

Foods with more yang, or contracted energy remain viable longer and can come from a greater distance than foods with more yin, or expansive energy. Sea salt and sea vegetables are examples. They are rich in contracted minerals and can come from the oceans around the world, provided these waters are within your hemisphere. Grains, especially with the outer husk attached, remain intact for a long time, even thousands of years, and can come from anywhere in your continent. Beans also travel well and can come from a similarly wide area. However, vegetables and fruits are more yin or expansive; they decompose more rapidly than grains and beans, and unless they are naturally dried or pickled, are best taken from your immediate area.

Changing with Our Environment

It is also important to adapt our cooking and eating to seasonal changes. The modern way of eating does not do this, as people eat pretty much the same diet throughout the year. High temperatures and bright sunshine produce a stronger charge of upward energy in the environment. Water evaporates more rapidly and plants become lush and expanded. Spring and summer are times of upward, expansive energy. Then toward the end of summer, energy starts to change, moving downward and inward. In colder and darker conditions, such as those of autumn and winter, downward or contracting energy is stronger.

How can we adapt to these changes? During spring and summer, we can make our diet lighter and fresher, meaning that we use less fire in cooking. We do not need as much fire in our cooking because fire is already there in the form of strong sunshine. When it is hot, we do not need warmth from our food. As we move into autumn and winter, with cooler temperatures and stronger downward energy, we make our food hearty and warming by using more fire in cooking.

As the seasons change, we also need to utilize the natural products of our environment. Our gardens are filled with vegetables and other foods during the spring and summer, so we can naturally eat plenty of fresh garden produce during these times. For example, summer is the time when corn is readily available, so it is fine to eat plenty of fresh corn in that season.

From season to season, atmospheric energy alternates as part of the daily cycle. Upward energy is stronger in the morning, while downward energy is stronger in the afternoon and evening. In order to eat in harmony with this cycle, breakfast should be light, not heavy. A breakfast of eggs and bacon is dense and heavy, and goes against the movement of energy. Breakfast grains can be cooked with more water, so that they become lighter and more easily digested. Dinner can include a greater number of side dishes, and we normally eat more in the evening, since at that time, atmospheric energy is more condensed and inward-moving. Lunch can also be quick and light, since at noon, atmospheric energy is very active and expansive. Quick light cooking, such as that in which we reheat leftovers, can be done at that time.

Respecting Human Needs

An important macrobiotic principle is to eat according to our distinctive needs as a species. Our teeth reveal the ideal proportion of foods in the human diet. We have thirty-two adult teeth. There are twenty molars and premolars. The word molar is a Latin word for "millstone," or the stones used to crush wheat and other grains into flour. These teeth are not suited for animal food, but for crushing or grinding grains, beans, seeds, and other tough plant fibers. There are also eight front incisors (from the Latin, "to cut") and these are well-suited for cutting vegetables. We also have four canine teeth. The canines can be used for animal food, not necessarily meat, but foods such as white-meat fish. The ideal proportion of foods as reflected in the teeth is five parts grain and other tough fibrous foods, two parts vegetables, and one part animal food. The ideal ratio between plant and animal food is seven to one.

The modern diet does not reflect this pattern. Rather than whole grains, meat or other types of animal food are the primary foods. Vegetables are used only as a garnish to the main course of animal food. Cereal grains are eaten almost as an afterthought, and are eaten in the form of white bread, white rolls, and other highly refined products. Refined bread or rolls are used simply as a vehicle to carry a hot dog, hamburger, or some other type of animal food. Grains are an incidental part of the modern diet.

Today, people are eating the opposite of what they should be eating. That is why so many health problems exist in the modern world. One of the clearest messages I received from the books of George Ohsawa was that plant-based diets are superior to animal-based diets. When Ohsawa presented that idea many years ago, Western doctors and nutritionists laughed. They believed that animal protein was superior to plant protein, and that cultures in which animal protein formed the basis of the diet were more advanced than cultures that relied on grains and other plant foods.

However, that view is changing. The vanguard of modern nutrition now agrees that plant-based diets are better for our health. If we compare the health patterns of people who are eating plant-based diets with those who are eating animal food, the grain- and vegetable-eaters have far lower rates of chronic disease. There is an exception to this of course. If you would like to eat animal food, it would be better for you to move to the Far North, above the Arctic Circle. Then you can eat plenty of animal food. But if you live in Houston, where it is a hundred degrees in the summer, then it is out of order to eat barbecued steak. It does not fulfill our biological needs nor does it make our condition harmonious with our environment.

Macrobiotics also recommends respecting dietary tradition. In the Bible we read, "give us this day our daily bread." Bread is symbolic of grain itself. Wheat, barley, and other grains were considered the staff of life. In the Far East, rice was considered the staple food, the staff of life. Native Americans respected corn as their staff of life. Wherever you look, no matter what your tradition is, if you go back far enough, you find that your ancestors were eating grains as their principal foods. They used local vegetables and beans as secondary foods. They were eating much less animal food than at present.

Nightshade vegetables, especially tomatoes and potatoes, were originally not a part of the diet in Europe. These vegetables were brought to Europe from Peru. The original Italian diet did not include tomato sauce. It was very close to a macrobiotic diet. Originally they did not use much meat, they used more seafood, because Italy is a peninsula. They did not use butter, but used olive oil in cooking. Instead of umeboshi plums, they used pickled olives. The basis of the diet was whole grain pasta and rice. As people abandoned these traditional eating patterns in favor of the modern diet, their rates of degenerative disease, especially heart disease and cancer, increased dramatically.

Food as Energy

The practice of macrobiotics is based on the understanding of food as energy. Electrons and protons are not solid particles, but condensed packets of energy. Everything is actually energy, everything is composed of vibration. There is no unchanging or fixed substance in the universe. Therefore, our understanding of food incorporates, but is not limited to, theories of modern nutrition. In modern nutrition, food is viewed as matter. In reality, there is an invisible quality to food (and to life itself) that cannot be measured scientifically. We must perceive that invisible quality directly through our intuition.

In macrobiotics, we employ a very simple tool for understanding the movement of energy. We understand food in terms of yin (expansion) and yang (contraction). All foods are made up of varying degrees of these two basic forces. We use this understanding to see how food affects us in a very dynamic and practical way. By understanding food as energy, we see that it affects not only our physical condition, but our mind, emotions, and even our spirituality. These invisible aspects of life are a function of the quality of energy we manifest.

If we eat a food such as steak, which is very yang or contracted, we are naturally attracted to foods with the opposite quality of energy. So we eat the steak with potatoes, alcohol, or a sugary dessert such as ice cream. All of these foods are extremely yin. In order to balance extremes, we have to add many things that we don't need. We wind up taking in excess fat, excess protein, excess carbohydrate, and excess water. Our body is constantly being challenged.

However, what happens when our main food is more balanced? If you look at a nutritional analysis of whole grains—brown rice, barley, millet, whole wheat—you discover that their ratio of minerals to protein and protein to carbohydrate approximates one to seven. Short grain brown rice comes closest to the one to seven ratio, that, nutritionally speaking, represents the balancing point between expansive and contractive energies on the planet. If you eat whole grains every day, your main foods are balanced in themselves. It is much easier to balance yin and yang in your diet as a whole. Eating whole grains as your primary food makes it much easier to maintain optimal nutritional and energetic balance.

Macrobiotics recommends that our foods be as natural as possible. Today, however, people are using poor quality table salt, treated city water, animal protein instead of plant protein, saturated animal fat instead of vegetable oil, chemically processed rather than organic foods, and plenty of simple sugars instead of complex carbohydrates. It is no wonder that modern people's health is suffering, because the quality of each of these nutritional factors is poor.

The understanding of food as energy can guide us not only in creating an optimal diet, but in the use of simple home remedies for the relief of illness. For example, suppose someone has a kidney stone. What type of energy does that represent, more expansive, yin energy or more condensed, yang energy? A kidney stone is condensed, something like hard, frozen energy. In order to offset that, we need to apply something with the opposite, activating energy. Should we apply heat or cold? We should apply heat. Heat will activate this frozen energy and make it melt and break down. A hot ginger compress can be applied for that purpose.

Fever represents the opposite type of energy. Fever is an example of hot, overactive energy. What would balance that? Something with cool, inert energy. Ice is too cold for this purpose. Ice is so cold that it makes the body contract, so that the excess that is trying to come out through the fever will, instead, be held inside. Something a little milder is needed. Also, our body is part of the animal world, so something from the plant kingdom helps to make balance. A simple macrobiotic remedy for fever is to apply a cabbage leaf or another leafy green directly to the forehead. Another remedy is to take raw tofu, which is cool and inert, mash it, and apply it to the forehead. This application, known as a *tofu plaster*, draws heat out of the body. It can lower a fever in a matter of minutes. The principle of energy balance can help you manage a variety of minor conditions at home without aspirin or other medications.

Dietary Diversity

Macrobiotics also teaches that we respect biodiversity, or the tremendous proliferation of life on earth. Many people are concerned with preserving the wealth of species on our planet because biodiversity is now being threatened by civilization. Many species, including those in tropical rain forests, are disappearing. Others are in danger. Scientists have discovered that amphibians such as frogs and salamanders are diminishing, perhaps because of ozone depletion or acid rain. The tiger, the symbol of power and beauty, is vanishing from the wild. However, in nature, biodiversity is the rule, not the exception. To reflect this in our eating, we need to practice what I call *dietary diversity*. There is a wide proliferation of life on earth, a wide range of species, and to translate that into our day to day eating, we need plenty of variety in our selection of foods, and also in our cooking methods. Macrobiotic eating is not narrow or strict. Through macrobiotics, we discover a wide range of healthful new foods.

We also need to respect the endless diversity of individual needs. Although we share certain fundamental things in common, each of us is different. If we are active, we should eat a certain way for physical activity. If we are sitting behind a desk, our diet should be somewhat different. Men and women also need to eat differently. Between men and women, who can eat more animal food? Men. Who can eat more raw salad and sweets? Women. Children and adults also need to eat differently. Babies are already yang—small and contracted—so their diets need to be more yin—soft and sweet-tasting, with little or no salt. If you have eaten plenty of animal food in the past, in order to restore balance, you need to base your diet on plant foods. Or if you have a health problem caused by your past way of eating, you can emphasize certain foods in order to offset that.

Benefits of Macrobiotics

What are the benefits of macrobiotic living? Eating this way can help us maintain optimal health and achieve longevity. People such as the Hunza in Kashmir, known for their good health and longevity, eat grains and vegetables as their main food. They were eating more or less a macrobiotic diet adapted to their mountainous terrain and climate. The first benefit of macrobiotic eating is physical health and longevity.

A second benefit is peace of mind. That peace of mind comes from the awareness that we are living and eating in harmony with the universe. We are living in harmony with the movement of energy. That is the source of inner peace. Our mind and emotions are very much conditioned by what we eat. If you feed your child plenty of sugar, what kind of mind or emotions result? Children become hyperactive or cry a lot, and become overly emotional. If we eat plenty of meat, what kind of mind and emotions are produced? We become aggressive or in the extreme, even violent. What happens when we eat plenty of nightshade vegetables such as tomatoes or potatoes? We become depressed. Incidentally, these vegetables have recently been found to contain nicotine. Nicotine is an addictive substance, and that may explain why many people find it difficult to stop eating these vegetables.

As your mind and emotions become more stable and peaceful, you naturally develop a sense of family and community. Modern values—such as competition, dog eat dog, survival of the fittest, etc.—have all arisen from a carnivorous diet. Grain-eating people develop a completely opposite view. Instead of seeing scarcity on the earth, we realize that we live in a universe of abundance. Rather than fighting over resources, the issue becomes how to share the tremendous natural wealth on our planet. Meat-eating tends to produce isolation, something like the lone hunter or lone wolf, rather than a sense of community. Hunters such as lions and hyenas are constantly fighting with each other. Grain-eaters develop a completely opposite way of thinking based on cooperation.

Meat-eating also leads to a more nomadic lifestyle, following the herd, and we tend to become unsettled, rather than stable or settled down. Grain-eating agricultural life is more stable, more settled. Which way of life encourages more stable family life? When the men are off hunting all season, or if the entire village has to constantly be on the move, it is difficult to maintain stability. Macrobiotic living strengthens our community and family life. People naturally desire to help and support each other. Through macrobiotics, you become friends with everyone. As we continue to eat this way, our concept of family expands to include all of humanity. We reconnect with our human family on planet earth.

Macrobiotic living can also help us gain spiritual understanding. Do you think it is easy to meditate if we eat hamburgers, or if our mind is very angry or upset, or if we are always stressed out? Or if we are eating sugar or drinking Coke all the time, so that our mind is often hyperactive and scattered, can we really stabilize and center our energy? These conditions make if very difficult to enter into deep, tranquil, and peaceful meditation. In order to allow spiritual energy to smoothly channel through us, and to use that energy, macrobiotic eating—grains and vegetables—is ideal. We should not forget that all great spiritual traditions included some form of dietary discipline. In the Orient, the cooking in Buddhist and Taoist monasteries was called *Shojin-Ryori*, or "cooking for spiritual development." These traditions were based on the understanding that food accelerates our spiritual consciousness. By selecting the proper food, we develop our spiritual quality. In these traditions, do you think animal food was a part of their diets? No. They were completely vegetarian. However, in traditional times, vegetarian eating, especially in cooler climates, meant eating cooked brown rice, daikon and other vegetables, tofu and bean products, etc., rather than a lot of raw fruit or salad.

Finally, as we achieve good health, peace of mind, a sense of family and community, and spiritual understanding, we gain the ability to play and have a big dream or adventure in this life. Macrobiotics is based on change or transmutation. In other words, we try to gain the ability to change things into their opposite according to our free will. So if we are experiencing difficulty, using macrobiotic understanding, we try to change that into pleasure or enjoyment. Or if we are experiencing sickness, we self-transform that into health. Or if the world is in danger of war, as our adventure, as our play, as our challenge, we transform that into peace. You can even gain the ability to transmute or transform any type of food into your health and vitality. In other words, you embrace your antagonist and turn it into your friend. As George Ohsawa said, ultimately there are no restrictions. The realization of total freedom, or the freedom to play endlessly in this infinite universe, is the ultimate benefit of macrobiotic living.

Source: This essay is from a lecture at the Macrobiotic Summer Conference in Poultney, Vermont, August, 1994.

2.
Yin and Yang in Social Organization

The most basic social relationship is that between a man and a woman. Men and women are complementary opposites, and are attracted to each other. Out of their union comes the social unit known as the family. Humanity exists because of the attraction and harmony between these opposite energies.

In society, there are two types of organization. One is based on the structure of the family, and is more natural. The other is based on artificial concepts. These opposite approaches to social organization have arisen because of differences in environment and food patterns, as we see in the following table:

Family-Style Organization	Conceptual Organization
Based on love and trust	Based on fear and distrust
Emphasis on natural harmony	Emphasis on conceptual regulation
Cooperation	Competition
Traditional	Modern
Flexible	Rigid
Monistic	Dualistic
Product of a plant-based diet	Product of a diet based on animal food

In the world of business, more rigid, conceptual models

of organization were adopted by Western countries, beginning in the early part of this century. On the other hand, Japanese businesses adopted a more family-style of organization.

After the Second World War, Japanese industry was completely destroyed. Now, the Japanese economy is second only to that of the United States. One reason for this success is the Japanese approach to management, in which a family-style of organization is is combined with modern business.

Another reason for their success is their more holistic approach to work. Modern assembly line manufacturing, for example, is fragmented and dehumanizing. A worker will spend the entire day performing the same task over and over, such as placing a weld in a car door. The inhumanity of the modern factory was portrayed in the 1930s in *Modern Times*, the classic film by Charlie Chaplin. Such fragmentation separates people from each other and from their natural creativity. It is hard for them to feel pride or accomplishment in their work.

The modern assembly line process was developed by Henry Ford. It is the product of a meat-centered diet. Ford visited meat packing plants in Chicago where fully automated, "disassembly lines," had been put into place. In these automated factories, living cows were turned into packaged meat products. Workers would perform the same task again and again for the entire day. Ford was so impressed with the efficiency of this method that he simply reversed the process, creating what became known as the "assembly line" approach to manufacturing.

The Japanese have a more holistic approach to production. Instead of isolated workers performing fragmented tasks, they use "production teams," in which teams of workers perform a variety of tasks. Workers are more connected to each other and to the process of production as a whole. They naturally feel a greater sense of pride and accomplishment in their work. Combined with their family style of organization, the team approach to production has enabled the Japanese to achieve staggering economic gains. This approach to work came from a culture in which grains and vegetables were the principal foods.

As more people shift away from animal food and toward a

diet of grains and vegetables, we can expect our orientation toward work to change. In the future, our approach to work will evolve in a more holistic and natural direction, and lead everyone toward greater self-realization and fulfillment.

Source: This essay is based on lectures at the East West Foundation in Boston.

Homeopathy and Chewing

Dr. Samuel Hahnemann, an 18th century German physician, was the founder of homeopathy. Hahnemann discovered that the more diluted a particular medicine was, the greater its potency. He called this phenomenon the law of infinitesimals. Thus, the most powerful homeopathic remedies are those which are so highly diluted that no molecules of the original substance are left; only the vibrational essence of the substance remains.

Macrobiotic healing is based on a similar concept. Macrobiotics begins with the premise that the most powerful medicine is our daily food. We activate the vibrational essence of food through cooking. Then, we dilute the food in our mouths through chewing. When we chew, we apply Hahnemann's law of infinitesimals: the more we chew, the more diluted—and the more powerful—the food becomes. Moreover, diluting food with saliva also makes the healing properties of this highly energized liquid available to us. Thorough chewing is thus essential to liberate the vibrational essences and healing powers of our daily foods.

3.
The Beauty of Rice Fields

One of the most profound experiences I have had took place a number of years ago on a clear October day in the mountains and rice fields that surround the city of Kyoto. During an afternoon walk on the outskirts of the city, I decided to stray from the main road onto one of the paths that led to a large clearing at the foot of a mountain. The plain was overflowing with fields of ripening rice, and as I continued walking, I found myself surrounded on all sides by acre after acre of golden grain. The sun was shining in a warm, late afternoon yellow and the sky was a crystal blue. The pine-studded mountains off in the distance were a brilliant green.

In this beautifully natural setting, everything seemed in perfect harmony—living, breathing, vibrant with the energy of heaven and earth. Underlying the feeling of peace, harmony, and serenity, which seemed to extend throughout the universe, was the deep sense of attraction and oneness I felt for the ripening rice.

The magnetism that I experienced so vividly that afternoon is a result of the natural attraction that human beings have for the vegetable kingdom, especially cereal grains. Without this attraction we literally would not exist, since without these primary foods, there would be no human life. However, as fundamental as it is, our attraction to cereal grains is only one of a countless number of complementary and antagonistic, or yin and yang relationships existing in nature.

The duality which bisects nature originates within the wholeness or oneness of the infinite universe, and comes into being when the oneness of the universe polarizes itself into two complementary and antagonistic forces, or yin and yang. This process is without beginning or end, and occurs in the form of a spiral, which is the most basic form of everything in the universe. The spiral of life flows continuous and unbroken through time and space. I could sense the vast dimensions of this spiral that day in the rice field. The rice, the sacred grain of Far Eastern peoples, gives itself, changes itself into human flesh and spirit. The rice, along with all other products of the vegetable kingdom, is in turn created by the sky, wind, earth, and water. These elemental forms are created by the aggregation of electrons, protons, and other particles that comprise the preatomic world. All of these worlds are alive with energy or spirit, and are the product of the everlasting and imperishable forces of centrifugality and centripetality, or yin and yang, that emanate continuously from the oneness of the infinite universe itself.

Humanity exists at the center of this universal spiral of life. Macrobiotics is the art of harmonizing these universal forces as they appear on earth. In this way, we move in the same direction as the spiral of life. Biologically, this condition of harmony is referred to as health, while psychologically, we refer to it as happiness. The macrobiotic way of life is based on the understanding of the order of the universe itself. It offers not only a common sense approach to personal health, but a fundamental method for the achievement of social harmony and peace.

I returned home energized and inspired. I realized that my experience in the rice field had brought me closer to an understanding of universal truth.

Source: This essay is adapted from Macrobiotic Cooking for Everyone, *Japan Publications, Tokyo and New York, 1980.*

4.
A Unifying Cosmology

Our study of macrobiotics, which will help lay the groundwork for the civilization of the future, is based on a view of life that encompasses the entire universe.

At the basis of this understanding is the logarithmic spiral of the universe. The logarithmic spiral, which appears throughout nature, reveals the mechanism of creation and the fundamental unity and interconnectedness of life. The spiral form enables us to unify all contradictions in science and other domains of thought.

A major problem confronting humanity is the split between science, or the study of the material world, and philosophy or religion, which have traditionally concerned themselves with the invisible worlds of mind, consciousness, and spirit. However, the notion that these domains are separate is an illusion. Both are within the spiral and are different appearances of the indivisible unity of life.

Throughout history, the separation between science and religion has erupted into conflict. During the Middle Ages, the church was the dominant power and science was still in its infancy. However, because theologians often interpreted biblical teachings in a dogmatic way, they were unable to embrace this newer field of knowledge. Witness the persecution of Galileo, Copernicus, and others who presented views that differed from those of the church.

In 19th century England, science and religion clashed as Darwin's scientific theory of evolution appeared and challenged the biblical account of creation. However, if we refer to the logarithmic spiral, we can see that these opposite views are actually complementary. The Book of Genesis describes the evolution or creation of the universe in terms of a seven-staged process, beginning with the absolute, undifferentiated world of God or infinity. This process continues through the worlds of polarization, or yin and yang (heaven and earth); energy or vibration (light and darkness); the preatomic world (the firmament); the world of elements (dry land and water); culminating in the appearance of plants, and then animals and man, as represented by Adam and Eve. Darwin was attempting to describe the process of change or transformation that occurred within the inner orbits of the spiral; more specifically, since the appearance of biological life on earth.

From the point of view of the unifying principle, as illustrated by the logarithmic spiral, we can understand that the theory of evoulution and the biblical account of creation are simply complementary ways of expressing the same thing. As the above example illustrates, the logarithmic spiral enables us to unify science and philosophy, West and East, modern and traditional understanding and lay the foundation for a more unified, planetary civilization.

Source: This essay is from lectures at the Kushi Institute in Boston.

5.
Diet and Behavior

In its structure and function, the brain and nervous system is a masterpiece of complementary balance. The cells in the nervous system, known as neurons, come in a variety of forms, but share the same basic structure. The sections of the neuron include branched dendrites, which receive incoming impulses; the yang or compact cell body, where impulses gather and are processed, and the yin, extended axon where impulses are dispatched to neighboring cells.

On the whole, each cell in the nervous system functions as a spiral made up of incoming and outgoing impulses and energy.

When nerve impulses arrive at the end point, or terminal of the axon, they travel across the synapse, a narrow space that separates the axons of nerve cells from the dendrites of others. When impulses reach the terminal, they stimulate the release of neurotransmitters, substances that determine the way that the message will affect the neighboring cell. More yang, activating transmitters cause nerve cells to become excited and generate impulses at a higher rate. More yin, inhibiting transmitters slow or block the production of nervous impulses.

Foods such as whole grains, beans, and vegetables rich in complex carbohydrates increase the brain's supply of serotonin, a more yin neurotransmitter that is believed to induce calm and relaxed mental states. Eggs and other animal food increase the levels of acetylcholine, another neurotransmitter. That may help explain why persons who consume grains and vegetables and little or no animal food often seem calm and even-tempered in comparison to persons who consume plenty of meat and other animal foods. The low levels of serotonin that result from a diet high in animal foods may contribute to impulsive behavior. In studies of prison inmates conducted in Finland, those with the most impulsive behavior patterns were found to have the lowest levels of metabolized serotonin in the spinal fluid when compared to non-impulsive prisoners and controls. The impulsive inmates were also found to have low blood sugar levels. The researchers found that 81 percent of repeat offenders had abnormally low blood sugar levels. Low levels of serotonin, together with low levels of blood sugar, characterized 84 percent of the repeat offenders studied.

Diet also affects the body's secretion of hormones, and these also influence behavior. In a study conducted at Yale, the intake of refined sugar was found to dramatically increase blood levels of adrenaline in children. In children who were tested after being given an amount of sugar equivalent to two cupcakes, levels of adrenaline increased ten times. Adrenaline, secreted by the adrenal glands during times of stress, initiates the "fight or flight" response. It produces such effects as rapid heartbeat, quick shallow breathing, and nervousness.

High adrenaline levels lead to anxiety and difficulty in thinking clearly. Parents often notice that children behave in an aggressive, hyperactive, and erratic manner after eating plenty of sugary foods, and this study offers a possible biochemical explanation for this reaction. Researchers are becoming aware that diet has a profound effect on the the brain and nervous system, and thus on our mental and emotional condition.

According to the National Institutes of Mental Health, about 5 percent of the American population suffers from major depressive illness. Milder forms of depression are much more common. Suicide is often the outcome of severe depression, and about 75,000 people commit suicide every year in the United States. Suicide is the second leading cause of death among men between the ages of twenty-five and forty-five, and the rate is increasing among young people.

Bouts of depression often occur in cycles. A bout of depression may last for one or two days or for several months or longer. Researchers have begun to observe a correlation between episodes of depression and natural rhythms such as the 24-hour daily cycle and the cycle of the seasons. Depression tends to be more severe in the afternoon and evening, and during the autumn and winter, times when the energy of the earth's atmosphere becomes more yang or condensed.

In many cases, depression is the by-product of a condition known as hypoglycemia, or low blood sugar. Hypoglycemia is produced by an extreme or unbalanced diet, especially the regular intake of cheese, chicken, eggs, and other forms of animal food. These more yang or contractive items cause the pancreas to become hard and tight, and inhibit its secretion of glucagon, or anti-insulin, the more yin pancreatic hormone that raises the level of glucose in the blood. When the pancreas becomes hard and tight, it cannot secrete glucagon properly, although insulin, the more yang hormone that lowers blood sugar, keeps being secreted. The result is hypoglycemia. Hypoglycemia creates the desire to consume sugar, soft drinks, chocolate, alcohol, or drugs, all of which raise the level of sugar in the blood.

The brain is utterly dependent on glucose for its functioning, and when a deficit arises, the higher brain centers, including those governing imagination and creativity, shut down in order to conserve more fundamental brain activity essential for survival. This produces a sinking feeling or a feeling of being boxed in by circumstances. A person becomes unable to imagine a solution to whatever problems he may be experiencing, and, because of a lack of blood sugar, may not have enough energy to change his circumstances. The result is depression and a sense of hopelessness.

The principle of yin and yang can help clarify the biochemistry of depression and other mood disorders. When the blood sugar becomes elevated (yin), the pancreas secretes insulin (yang), in order to make balance. In the brain, production of more yang neurotransmitters—those involved in arousal and motor activity—is stepped up. Conversely, when blood sugar becomes low (yang), the pancreas reduces the output of insulin, while accelerating production of glucagon (yin). In the brain, production of activating neurotransmitters is reduced, in some cases, to the point of undersupply. The resulting shortage can lead to depression.

A naturally balanced, macrobiotic diet can help correct these imbalances in the internal chemistry of the body. A diet based on complex carbohydrates, such as those in whole grains, beans, and fresh local vegetables helps stabilize the metabolism of glucose, and can help relieve conditions such as depression, fear, and anxiety. Mind and body are one. The application of diet to the relief of mood disorders represents a new frontier in the field of psychology.

Blood sugar imbalances also play an important role in schizophrenia, a more severe form of mental illness. Chronic low blood sugar leads to cravings for refined sugar, alcohol, chocolate, drugs, and other extreme forms of yin. The continual intake of extreme yin items can cause the cells of the brain and nervous system to become chronically expanded, producing an eventual deterioration of mental functioning. The result can be schizophrenia.

Our mental processes depend on the brain's ability to concentrate and simplify information. This process is more yang. In *The Healing Brain*, Robert Ornstein and David Sobel describe this process as follows:

> Since the world is constantly changing, the brain is flooded with information. How would it know which of all these changes are important and which are irrelevant? A strategy emerged in which the brain and nervous system evolved to radically reduce and limit the information transmitted to the brain.
> The nervous system organizes information so that a few actions, the appropriate actions, can take place. Much of the intricate network of receptors, ganglia, and analysis cells in the cortex serve to simplify. Senses select only a few meaningful elements from all the stimuli that reach us, organize them into the most likely occurrence, and remember only a small organized sample of what has occurred.

When brain cells become chronically yin or expanded,

they easily become overly sensitive to yang stimuli, including activating neurotransmitters such as dopamine. According to a popular hypothesis, oversensitivity to this neurotransmitter produces chronic hyper-stimulation in the brain. The patient becomes hypersensitive to stimulation from the immediate environment and loses touch with vibrations coming from greater distances. This leads to cognitive overload and a decline in more refined thinking abilities. A person in this condition has difficulty organizing the world by going beyond the immediate information he receives.

Coordinating the varied functions of the brain requires strong yang, or centripetal power. Ornstein and Sobel describe these varied functions as follows:

> The brain is divided into very many independent and well-defined areas, each of which possesses a rich concentration of certain abilities. In this view, which is becoming more and more established, the brain is seen not as a single organ, but as a collage of different and independent systems, each of which contains component abilities.

In schizophrenia, the yang power of coordination and control breaks down. The various centers of the brain may start to act independently. The spiral of coordination begins to spin out of control. This is due to an overly yin condition in the brain and nerve cells. People with schizophrenia often show signs of excess sugar consumption. Refined sugar disrupts the balance of vitamins and minerals in the body. A common symptom of schizophrenia is numerous white spots on the fingernails, a sign of mineral deficiency resulting from the repeated consumption of simple sugar. Many schizophrenics also have a sweet odor on their breath, also the result of consuming sugar. A variety of mineral deficiencies and imbalances are also common, especially deficiencies in zinc, manganese, magnesium, and sodium, and these result primarily from the repeated consumption of sugar.

The regular intake of simple sugars also depletes B-complex vitamins that are necessary to smooth mental functioning. More than fifty years ago, it was discovered that vitamin B deficiencies were related to mental illness. About 10 percent of the people who were diagnosed with schizophrenia and committed to mental hospitals in the South were found to be suffering from pellagra, a vitamin B deficiency. When they were placed on corrective diets, their previously diagnosed "schizophrenia" cleared up.

A naturally balanced, macrobiotic diet, rich in B vitamins, minerals, complex carbohydrates, and other essential nutrients, could help many patients with schizophrenia. Restoring the brain and nervous system to a more normal balance of yin and yang is the first step toward the recovery from mental illness.

Source: This essay is from personal notes and lectures, including research for the book, Crime and Diet, *Japan Publications, Tokyo and New York, 1987.*

Attraction and Repulsion

Hammering a nail into wood offers an example of attraction and repulsion. Both the nail and the wood are solid objects (yang) and therefore repel each other. In order to drive the nail into the wood, we must overcome this repulsion. Hammering causes the nail to become extremely yang. The wood then becomes yin in relation to it, thus allowing the nail to penetrate (opposites attract). When similar things repel one another, we call that "friction" or "resistance"; when opposites attract, we refer to that as "harmony" or "acceptance."

6.
Conversations with T. Colin Campbell

"Whoever gives these things [food] no consideration, and is ignorant of them, how can he understand the diseases of man?"
—Hippocrates

On a snowy morning in December, 1992, I boarded a bus bound for Ithaca, New York. Friends in Ithaca had invited me to lecture in their city, and in spite of the winter storm, we decided to go ahead with our plan. As it turned out, the city of Ithaca did not receive much snowfall, although the area around it did. An enthusiastic group turned out for the lectures and other educational events held over the weekend.

During the visit, a friend mentioned that Dr. T. Colin Campbell, the well-known diet and health researcher, was a neighbor of hers. Dr. Campbell is a professor at Cornell University, and principal author of the landmark China Health Study. The China Health Study made headlines in June, 1990, after preliminary results were published by Cornell University Press. This huge epidemiological study, conducted in association with the Chinese government, added substantial weight to the evidence supporting the advantages of eating a diet based on whole grains, vegetables, beans, and other plant foods.

I mentioned to my friend that I very much wanted to meet Dr. Campbell. She graciously called him and mentioned my request. In spite of a tight schedule, he said he would have time the following day to meet with me. The meeting took place at his home. Paula Dore, a friend from Ithaca, accompanied me to the meeting.

After shaking hands, Dr. Campbell led us into his living room. He is a soft-spoken, unassuming man. As we sat down, I thanked him for his pioneering research. What followed was an animated discussion about the need for continuing research and education on diet and health.

I started by describing the role macrobiotic education has played in furthering dietary awareness in the United States and abroad. I mentioned the pioneering role that macrobiotic education has played in starting the natural food and health revolutions. We then discussed the need for formal research on the role of diet in the prevention of and recovery from cancer and other chronic diseases.

Dr. Campbell told me that the findings of the China Health Study were being taken very seriously in China, Indonesia, and other Asian countries, and in some cases, national agricultural and dietary policies are now being based on its findings. The meeting concluded with an affirmation of our mutual interest in working together.

Soon afterward, Dr. Campbell sent me two articles that he was preparing for publication. In the accompanying letter he stated:

> I enclose the two manuscripts that I wrote for a book to be co-edited by Denis Burkitt and Norman Temple that I spoke to you about while you were here.
>
> In one chapter, I critiqued the contemporary research focused on the so-called dietary guidelines and, with published data, found that these recommendations, as conventionally practiced, are likely to do little or nothing. In the second chapter, I and Junshi Chen summarized the findings from our China project to present evidence showing, from many perspectives, that comprehensive disease prevention will come only if major adjustment of the animal/plant foods ratio is changed.

In these articles, Dr. Campbell elaborated on the findings of the China Health Study, especially in regard to the current preoccupation with the role of dietary fat in causing disease. In his view, dietary guidelines recommending a reduction of fat to 30 percent of total calories divert people from the more urgent need to make comprehensive dietary changes, and have little or no effect on lowering the risk of cancer and other chronic diseases.

Interest in the relationship between dietary fat and cancer dates back to the beginning of modern scientific medicine. In 1849, John Hughes Bennet, a professor of clinical medicine and author of a standard textbook on medicine in Britain, stated that "the circumstances which diminish obesity, and a tendency toward the formation of fat, would seem a priori to be opposed to the cancerous tendency."

Much of the evidence linking high fat intakes with breast and other forms of cancer comes from international correlation studies in which populations with high fat intakes were found to have a high rate of these diseases, while populations with the lowest fat intakes were found to have low or nonexistent rates. These findings are supported by animal studies showing that a high intake of fat promotes the development of tumors. However, these findings have not held up in dietary intervention studies, such as the Women's Health Trial and the Nurses Health Study, in which groups of women were placed on low-fat diets in order to determine whether or not lowering the intake of fat reduced the incidence of breast cancer. Unlike population and animal studies, these trials have failed to show a relationship between dietary fat and breast cancer.

According to Dr. Campbell, dietary fat is only one among other factors influencing the development of breast and other forms of cancer. The intake of animal protein may be just as important. When a "low-fat" diet is put into practice, most people, including the subjects in these studies, simply switch to lower fat varieties of animal food, for example, from beef to chicken, and from whole fat dairy products to "low-fat" varieties. As a result, their intake of animal protein remains at its already high level, or may actually increase. (For the first time in history, per capita consumption of chicken is now higher than that of beef. Chicken has replaced red meat as the leading form of animal food consumed in the U.S., largely as the result of public health guidelines that recommend eating more low-fat animal foods.)

There is evidence that the intake of animal protein has a significant influence on the development of cancer. In population studies, countries with high fat intakes also have high intakes of animal protein, and their intake of protein may be an important factor in their high cancer rate. At the same time, when a person adopts a low-fat diet, he or she will usually reduce fat intake by several percentage points only, while failing to increase the consumption of whole grains, fresh vegetables, beans, sea vegetables, and other plant foods that have cancer-inhibiting properties. As a result, people receive little or no preventive benefit from such a minor change in diet.

Paralleling the focus on dietary fat is the growing interest in the cancer-inhibiting potential of single nutrients. There are now 500 to 2,000 natural chemical substances, found mostly in plant foods, that are believed to "chemoprevent" cancer. For example, brown rice, whole wheat, barley, and other whole cereal grains have been found to contain substances known as protease inhibitors that are believed to suppress the action of proteases, enzymes suspected of promoting cancer. Protease inhibitors may also interfere with the activity of oncogenes, which under certain circumstances, are thought to stimulate normal cells to turn cancerous. Moreover, natural phytoestrogens, found in whole grains and soybean products, such as tofu, may inhibit the development of breast cancers. Researchers in England hypothesize that these compounds seem to work in the same way as tamoxifen, a drug that has been used in conventional therapy.

Miso, a fermented soybean paste, has long been associated with cancer prevention. A diet rich in soyfoods, especially miso soup, produces genistein, a natural compound that inhibits the growth of new blood vessels that feed tumors. Researchers from Children's University Hospital in Heidelberg, Germany, discovered that genistein also blocked cancer cells from multiplying and could have significant implications for the prevention and treatment of solid malignancies, including those of the brain, breast, and prostate.

Beta-carotene, a precursor to vitamin A, and other carotenoid pigments found in orange-yellow and dark leafy green vegetables, have also been shown to have cancer-inhibiting properties. Studies have also shown that cruciferous vegetables, such as cabbage, broccoli, cauliflower, turnips, and Brussels sprouts, contain numerous cancer-inhibiting substances, including indoles, chlorophyll, vitamin C, carotenoids, dithiolthiones, and glucosinolates, that are believed to be potent anti-cancer agents. Moreover, researchers have begun to identify numerous substances in sea vegetables that seem to protect against cancer.

Currently, about seventeen nutrient supplement trials are underway in which a small number of compounds are being tested in over 100,000 subjects. The participants in these studies are consuming their usual diets but taking these substances in supplement form. However, as with the failure of "minimalist" studies that focus only on fat intake, Dr. Campbell predicts that these supplement trials will fail to show a reduced risk of cancer. One or two isolated compounds will not be sufficient to overcome the overall negative effect of an unbalanced diet.

Dr. Campbell's views are strikingly similar to those of macrobiotic educators. In macrobiotic thinking, health or sickness result from the overall dietary pattern, and not from isolated components of the diet. To prevent chronic disease, a more total dietary change is necessary. Rather than isolating the cancer-inhibiting substances in grains, vegetables, beans, sea vegetables, and other plant foods, and taking these as supplements, macrobiotics recommends eating these foods in their whole form. The key to cancer prevention lies in eating whole natural foods, not in using dietary supplements or eating low-fat animal products.

In order for diet to have a genuinely preventive effect, Dr. Campbell suggests it may be necessary to reduce the consumption of fat to around 10 to 15 percent of caloric intake. For someone to get their fat intake down to this level, it is necessary to change the overall ratio of plant to animal food in the diet. Of necessity, a diet of 10 to 15 percent fat would require a substantial increase in the intake of whole grains, beans, vegetables, and other plant foods. Animal foods would become occasional supplements in an essentially plant-based diet. In his writings, Dr. Campbell returns again and again to this theme: researchers should investigate the preventive potential of a total readjustment of the animal to plant food ratio in the diet, rather than looking simply at a reduction in dietary fat or the inclusion of dietary supplements.

After years of study, Dr. Campbell has arrived at what George Ohsawa referred to as a "dialectical" understanding of nutrition, or an awareness of yin and yang, or complementary opposites in the realm of food and health. By drawing attention to the superiority of plant-based diets, he is essentially calling for a total reevaluation of modern nutrition. Coming from a realm dominated by analytical and partial thinking, his comprehensive views on diet and health are like a breath of fresh air.

According to the President's Cancer Panel, diet is the single largest cause of cancer. Despite the investment of billions of dollars in research and enormous effort, the rate of cancer is 18 percent higher today that it was in 1971, the year Richard Nixon launched the "War on Cancer." According to a study published in the *Journal of the American Medical Association*, a white male in his forties has twice the risk of developing cancer as his grandfather did, and a white female of the same age has a 150 percent greater chance of developing cancer as her grandmother did. The upward trend in cancer incidence has occurred even when the effects of smoking, the decline in heart disease, and the aging of the population are accounted for.

Currently, one-third of all Americans will develop cancer during their lifetime; by the year 2000, cancer will surpass heart disease as the leading cause of death in the United States. Given these statistics and the trail of human suffering caused by this disease, Dr. Campbell's and the macrobiotic message on diet and health could not be more timely.

Source: This essay is from personal notes and lectures.

7.
Teaching Macrobiotics in Southern California

On the night before my departure for California in March, 1993, a winter storm blew into the Berkshires. I got up before dawn and looked out the window. Snow was still falling.

I was traveling West to begin the Kushi Institute Extension (KIX) in Southern California. Since 1990, K.I. Extensions had started in Toronto, New York City, Philadelphia, Chicago, Cleveland, Dallas, and San Francisco. The Extension Program was started in order to bring comprehensive macrobiotic studies to people in different parts of the United States and Canada. The KIX program makes it possible for people around the country to pursue in-depth macrobiotic studies without having to travel to an established center. This was my second trip to California since the beginning of the year; a month before I had traveled to San Francisco to begin the K.I. Extension there.

I was traveling with Carry Wolf, a teacher at the K.I. in Becket. Carry was scheduled to present cooking classes as a part of the weekend.

That evening, a macrobiotic dinner and public lecture took place at the home of one of the students. About fifty people came, including many who were enrolled in the K.I. They had come from San Diego, Santa Barbara, Los Angeles, and other communities throughout Southern California.

After dinner, I spoke about macrobiotic healing, focusing on the use of food as medicine. I explained how an understanding of yin and yang and the energy of food is essential for genuine health and healing. I also mentioned a recent study in the *New England Journal of Medicine* in which researchers discovered that one-third of all Americans are using alternative healing methods. According to the study, alternative health care is now a $14-billion industry.

The K.I. session got underway on the following morning with Carry's cooking class. About twenty-five people are enrolled in the program. Classes are presented one weekend a month for ten months, and cover the same subjects—Order of the Universe, Macrobiotic Cooking, Oriental Diagnosis, Macrobiotic Health Care, and Shiatsu—that are presented in the Level I program in Becket. Many of the students had been practicing macrobiotics for some time and were familiar with the basic principles. Others were new to the macrobiotic way of life.

The cooking class focused on whole grains. Carry explained how to present a variety of healthful and delicious whole grain dishes, and talked about her experiences teaching and practicing macrobiotics in America and Europe. After lunch, I taught the class on the Order of the Universe. I explained how the principle of yin and yang is the basis for achieving health and happiness, and how it is found in all of the world's great spiritual, religious, and philosophical teachings, from the I Ching to the teachings of Jesus, and from the Old Testament to the teachings of Buddhism.

We used as examples quotations from the world's great spiritual and philosophical classics. For example, in Genesis, Chapter 1 we read of the polarization of one infinity, or God, into two complementary yet opposite energies:

In the beginning, God created the heaven and the earth.

The understanding of the law of change, especially the continual cycling between opposite states, is clearly expressed in Ecclesiastes, Chapter 1:

One Generation passeth away, and another generation cometh; but the earth abideth forever.
The sun also ariseth, and the sun goeth down, and

hasteth to his place where he arose.

The wind goeth toward the south, and turneth about unto the north; it whirleth about continually, and the wind returneth again according to his circuits.

All the rivers run into the sea; yet the sea is not full; unto the place from whence the rivers come, thither they return again.

In St. Matthew, Chapter 19, Jesus talks about the transformation of yin into yang and yang into yin:

But many that are first shall be last; and the last shall be first.

In the opening lines of the Nihon-Shoki, or Chronicles of Japan, compiled in the 8th century, we read of an account of creation that, like the account in Genesis, describes the polarization of the universe into heaven and earth, or yin and yang:

Of old, Heaven and Earth were not yet separated, and the In and Yo [yin and yang] not yet divided. They formed a chaotic mass like an egg which was of obscurely defined limits and contained seeds.

The purer and clearer part was thinly drawn out, and formed Heaven, while the heavier and grosser element settled down and became Earth.

The finer element easily became a united body, but the consolidation of the heavy and gross element was accomplished with difficulty.

Heaven was therefore formed first, and Earth was established subsequently.

Thereafter Divine Beings were produced between them.

Buddha's teachings evidence a clear understanding of the ephemerality of life and the constancy of change. In a farewell to his disciples he said:

My disciples, my end is approaching, our parting is near, but do not lament. Life is ever changing; none can escape the dissolution of the body. This I am now to manifest by my own death, my body falling apart like a decaying cart.

Do not vainly lament, but do wonder at the rule of transiency and learn from it the emptiness of human life. Do not cherish the unworthy desire that the changeable might become unchanging.

A similar understanding can be found in the sayings of Heraclitus, a pre-Socratic Greek philosopher:

> Immortals become mortals, mortals become immortals; they live in each other's death and die in each other's life. The universe throws apart and then brings together again; it advances and retires. Everything flows and nothing abides; everything gives way and nothing stays fixed. You cannot step twice into the same river, for other waters and yet others go ever flowing on.

In China, the teachings of Lao Tsu demonstrated a deep understanding of the order of the universe, or yin and yang. Lao Tsu's understanding is expressed clearly in the Tao Teh Ching, a small book composed of eighty-one poetic verses:

> In fact, for all things there is a time for going ahead and a time for following behind;
> A time for slow breathing and a time for fast breathing;
> A time to grow in strength and a time for decay;
> A time to be up and a time to be down.
>
> Difficult and easy complement each other.
> Long and short exhibit each other.
> High and low set measure to each other.
> Voice and sound harmonize each other.

Following our review of these and other historical expressions of the order of the universe, we studied the principle of commonness and difference. We began by listing the universal, common factors that are shared by all things. We discussed how even though all things share the same origin in the universe and the same process of change, they are at the same time completely unique. The principle of commonness and difference illustrates the macrobiotic principle that every front has a back, and every back has a front.

We then applied this principle to diet. I explained how the standard macrobiotic diet is derived from the common factors that all people share, such as a common environment on earth, a similar body structure, and common cultural traditions of grain and vegetable eating. The historical expressions of the order of the universe cited above, all of which share a universal common understanding, are the product of humanity's traditional diet of grains and vegetables. We then studied some of the ways in which the the macrobiotic diet can be modified to suit individual differences, such as those resulting from differences in climate, environment, age, sex, physical condition, level of activity, and personal tastes and desires. We also discussed how each of the historical expressions cited above was the product of the unique time, place, and environment in which it appeared, and that is why each one expresses the order of the universe in a different way.

On the second day, we delved further into our exploration of the order of the universe. We classified a variety of things into yin and yang, including general tendencies, foods, and types of people. The students participated actively in the group discussions and asked many questions. The weekend ended with a group meditation in which we joined hands and projected an image of health and peace throughout the world.

Source: This essay is from personal notes and lectures.

8.
Relativity

Suppose there are three cars driving on a road, all moving at different speeds in the same direction. If you are in the last car, the two cars in front of you appear to be moving in the opposite direction from you, one at a faster and the other at a slower rate. If you are in the lead car, the two cars that are behind you also appear to be moving away from you. If you continue at the same speed, they will eventually disappear behind you. If you are in the middle car, the lead car seems to be moving away from you in one direction (forward), while the last car is moving away from in the opposite direction. When seen from above, however, all of the cars seem to be moving at in the same direction but at different rates of speed. What we perceive as truth is always relative and dependent upon our point of view.

Yin and yang is the study of relative motion. Whether we judge something as more yin or more yang depends entirely upon our point of view. When you say that tomatoes are yin, they are yin only in relation to other things, such as squash and carrots. They also contain yang factors as well. If something were yin only, that would mean it was composed of pure expanding energy and thus would not exist. If something were yang only, it would contract infinitely and disappear. Both yin and yang are present in all things.

For example, yin and yang manifest in the continual cycling of day and night and the seasons. However, these cycles always appear in a relative form. When it is daytime in Boston, it is nighttime in Japan. When it is summer in Paris, it is winter in Buenos Aires.

There is also a tremendous daily and seasonal relativity existing along the earth's north/south axis. At the North Pole, there is no distinction between the days and the seasons. There is only a continual day that lasts for about six months during the summer, and a continual night that lasts for six months during winter. Here, day is equivalent to summer and night is equivalent to winter.

At the Arctic Circle (about 65 degrees north), there is no perpetual brightness or darkness, just very long days during the summer, and long nights in the winter. In the temperate zones, the two Polar seasons differentiate into four distinct seasons, with the days becoming longer in the summer, and shorter in winter. In the tropical zones, there is little variation in the length of day and night; night follows day at almost the same hour throughout the year. Also, in most tropical regions, there are only two distinct seasons during the year.

We should always be careful about believing that relative phenomena are "absolutely true." The scientific method, for example, is highly relative and changeable. There is no such thing as an "exact" science in our relative world. However, when you went to school, you were taught that one plus one is equal to two. That was not presented as a possibility, but as an absolute truth. If you did not agree with that equation, you were judged "wrong." One plus one may not always equal two; other answers may be equally correct.

When evaluating a theory or hypothesis, keep in mind that anything that can be weighed, measured, seen, imagined, or conceived of is a relative phenomenon. Scientific theories are themselves only approximations or guesses about the nature of reality and should not be mistaken for absolute or unchanging principles. The scientific "laws" of one generation are often outmoded by the next. The scientific method itself is only one way of looking at the world. There are other, complementary ways of understanding reality that are equally valid.

Source: This essay is from personal notes and lectures.

9.
Reflections on the Philosopher's Stone

"It is premature to reduce the vital process to the quite insufficiently developed conceptions of 19th and even 20th century physics and chemistry."

—L. de Broglie

The takeoff from Hartford was smooth and trouble-free. The 737 turned out over the Atlantic and headed south. The weather was rainy and the temperature mild for early December. After a brief stop in Charlotte, I boarded the forty-minute connecting flight to Atlanta. This was my third visit to Atlanta for lectures since 1984. Following Atlanta, I was scheduled to return to Charlotte for several days of teaching.

During the flight, I reflected on the book I just finished editing. Titled *The Philosopher's Stone*, it is based on Michio Kushi's lectures on alchemy and transmutation. According to legend, the philosopher's stone was the mysterious element used by medieval alchemists to transmute base metals into gold. To me, the philosopher's stone symbolizes the invisible law that produces all of the changes in the universe, including the transmutation of one element into another.

Transmutation has intrigued me since the beginning of my macrobiotic practice over twenty years ago. Much of the early macrobiotic literature contained references to the work of Louis Kervran, George Ohsawa, and others in the field of transmutation. Kervran, a French biochemist, discovered the transmutation of sodium into potassium in French workers in the Sahara. His findings were summarized in the book, *Biological Transmutations* (Happiness Press, 1987). George Ohsawa worked with Kervran and devoted the later years of his life to proving transmutation in the laboratory. In my thinking, transmutation offers proof of the mutability of the material world, and is at the core of the macrobiotic philosophy of change.

Writing in *Biological Transmutations*, Kervran describes the relationship between transmutation and modern chemistry and physics:

> The serious error of scientists consists in their saying that reactions occurring in living matter are solely chemical reactions, that chemistry can and must explain life. That is why in science we find such terms as "biochemistry." It is certain that a great number of manifestations of life are produced by chemical reactions. But the belief that there is only chemical reaction and that every observation must be explained in terms of a chemical reaction, is false. One of the purposes of this book is to show that matter has a property heretofore unseen, a property which is neither chemistry nor nuclear physics in its present state. In other words, the laws of chemistry are not on trial here. The error of numerous chemists and biochemists lies in their desire to apply the laws of chemistry at any cost, with unverified assertions, in a field where chemistry is not always applicable. In the final phase the result might be "chemistry," but only as a consequence of the unperceived phenomenon of transmutation.

When I visited Prague in 1990, friends took me to a section of the city called "Alchemists' Row." It is a narrow street on either side of which are curious tiny houses. Our guide explained that these houses were where medieval alchemists had lived and conducted their experiments. Prague was one of the centers of medieval European alchemy. The tiny houses on Alchemists' Row now serve as boutiques and gift shops for tourists.

Over the years, Michio Kushi has lectured on transmutation, and transcripts of these lectures were published in his seminar reports. Michio worked with Ohsawa and Kervran on transmutation experiments in New York and Cambridge. When I edited Michio's book *Other Dimensions: Exploring the Unexplained* (Avery, 1992), I included a chapter on transmutation. I have also lectured on the macrobiotic view of transmutation at the East West Foundation in Boston, and later as a part of the Kushi Institute's Level III program in Becket.

More recently, Michio announced that a group of scientists at a university in Texas had achieved the transmutation of carbon into iron, using Ohsawa's pioneering experiments as a guide. Michio also announced that he was planning to introduce this transmutation to industry in the hope of perfecting a method for the mass production of steel. As he states in *The Philosopher's Stone,* transmutation could be the key to changing industrial civilization and solving the global environmental crisis.

As the plane landed in Atlanta, my thoughts came back to the task at hand. I was met at the airport by Fred Rueff. Fred and his wife Marsha had started macrobiotics nine months before. Originally from Basel, Switzerland, Fred had undergone a triple bypass and had changed his diet to avoid a recurrence of his condition. With the help of Dr. Dean Ornish, Fred eliminated animal food and began to eat whole grains and vegetables. He eventually adopted a macrobiotic diet, and in nine months, the fat content of his body went from 12 to 8 percent. He explained that he was exercising on a regular basis and felt better than he had in years—an example of personal transmutation!

Following the weekend in Atlanta, I returned to Charlotte. I was met at the airport by Michel Matsuda. I first met Michel twenty years before in Boston, when both of us were studying with Michio and living in a macrobiotic student house. When Wendy and I visited Japan in 1978, Michel helped us get settled in Kyoto, his home city. Michel and his wife Libby, who is originally from Ireland, now run a macrobiotic study center in Charlotte. Aside from being a student of macrobiotics for the past thirty-five years, Michel is also a skilled acupuncturist. His practice in Charlotte is now quite active.

After leaving the airport, Michel and I went to a Japanese restaurant not far from his home. I mentioned the recent developments with atomic transmutation. Michel told me that he had been involved in transmutation research in Kyoto in the mid-Sixties. He led a group of young students, known as the *Circle of Seven* (named after Kurosawa's *Seven Samurai*) in the study and practice of transmutation. The group, inspired by the work of George Ohsawa and his associates, met weekly in an abandoned textile warehouse in Kyoto. The group started out with seven members, and eventually grew to include several dozen.

In June, 1964, Ohsawa achieved the transmutation of sodium into potassium (with the addition of oxygen) in the laboratory, under low temperature, pressure, and energy. He later achieved the transmutation of carbon into iron (with the addition of oxygen) under similar conditions. These discoveries challenge the prevailing notion that elements are fixed and separate, and change into each other only under very extreme circumstances, such as in a particle accelerator, during a thermonuclear reaction, or in the sun.

Inspired by Mr. Ohsawa's results, the Circle of Seven met weekly from 1965 to 1967. According to Michel, after much trial and error, they achieved the low-energy transmutation of carbon into iron. For Michel, these times were the most exciting in his thirty-five years of macrobiotic practice. He gave me the addresses of several member of the Circle of Seven after I expressed interest in writing to them for more information about their experiences.

In 1978, the U.S. Army commissioned a report on biological transmutations. The report concluded:

> Two investigators, Kervran and Komaki [an associate of George Ohsawa's], have been recently nominated for a joint Nobel prize for their work involving experimental proof that elemental transmutations were occurring in life organisms. Elements which were definitely proven to have been transformed were sodium (to magnesium), potassium (to calcium), and manganese (to iron). Actually, ob-

servations have been made for almost 200 years that elemental transmutations were occurring, but little credence was given to them because they resembled alchemy—a relic of the middle ages.

Modern physics and chemistry were born in the laboratories of the medieval alchemists. However, the quest for the philosopher's stone took a destructive turn in the twentieth century. In place of the peaceful, natural methods employed by ancient alchemists, modern researchers began to utilize violent and destructive methods to achieve transmutation.

In 1920, Rutherford changed nitrogen into hydrogen and oxygen by bombarding nitrogen atoms with subatomic alpha particles. Ten years later, Ernest Lawrence invented a device called the cyclotron in which atomic particles were accelerated with high energy and used to "smash" target atoms. In 1932, scientists discovered that neutrons could be used as "bullets" to smash atoms, and in 1939, the nucleus of uranium was "bombarded" with free neutrons, causing it to "split" and release energy. In 1942, Enrico Fermi at the University of Chicago used this discovery to achieve a chain reaction, and soon afterward, Oppenheimer and other researchers in the Manhattan Project used these discoveries to build the first atomic bomb.

After World War II, scientists used these discoveries to pursue nuclear fusion. Using an atomic bomb, they forced two atoms of hydrogen to fuse and form an atom of helium, releasing tremendous energy in the process. This led to the development of the thermonuclear, or hydrogen bomb. In 1953, the United States and the Soviet Union began to actively manufacture these weapons of mass destruction. Since then, nuclear weapons technology has spread around the globe. According to *Newsweek*, twenty-five nations have, or may soon have, nuclear weapons. The disposal of nuclear waste is also a gigantic problem. The U.S. Government recently revealed that it stores 33.5 metric tons of deadly radioactive plutonium in six states. Many of the storage facilities for nuclear waste are old and deteriorating rapidly. As we can see, the modern scientific pursuit of the ancient dream of the alchemists has led to a situation that threatens both humanity and the environment.

The discovery of peaceful, natural transmutation offers an alternative to these destructive methods. Atomic transmutation can be achieved under natural conditions without having to attack and destroy atoms. The work of George Ohsawa, Louis Kervran, Michio Kushi, the members of the Circle of Seven, and other pioneers in peaceful, natural transmutation have shown that the world of matter is not fixed and static, but dynamic and changing. These discoveries could revolutionize science and open the door to a new era for humanity. If this knowledge is properly understood and applied, the age-old quest for the philosopher's stone will contribute to an age of peace and prosperity. The transmutation of the atom is thus a metaphor for the transmutation of society itself.

Source: This essay appeared in MacroNews, *Philadelphia, Pa., Spring, 1994.*

Movement and Rest

In the macrobiotic classification, yang is activity, yin is rest. We can use a simple windup toy to illustrate this. When you wind the key, you are making the toy more yang. The tighter you wind the key, the more yang it becomes. When you release the key, this stored yang causes the toy to move. The toy will keep moving until its supply of yang is exhausted. Once the key is completely unwound (yin), the toy no longer moves and comes to a stop. In order to get it to move again, you must make it more yang.

10.
Seminars in Belgium and France

The East West Center in Antwerp has been active for over fifteen years. It was my first stop on a ten-day trip to Europe in February, 1994. The Center houses a spacious and well-stocked natural food store, managed by George van Wesenbeck, a friend from Boston, as well as offices and classrooms for lectures and cooking classes.

On the following day, Luc de Cuyper, the manager of the East West Center, showed me several of the Center's new educational programs, including regular backpacking tours to Spain, Portugal, Poland, and other places in Europe. The backpackers took macrobiotic foods and camped out during the tours. The program looked like great fun.

Luc had arranged a lecture that evening. Before the lecture, he and I joined Frans Copers, another friend from Boston who now manages a macrobiotic Shiatsu center in Ghent, at a Japanese natural food restaurant. Frans explained that awareness of diet was increasing in Belgium. He showed me an article published in *Knack*, a popular magazine in Belgium on the relationship between animal fats, and especially dairy foods, on heart disease and cancer. The article featured an interview with Dr. Hugo Kesteloot, a cardiologist and epidemiologist at the University of Leuven. Frans translated the following passage from the article:

If you think that progress in modern medicine plays an

important role in the decrease of cardiovascular mortality, Professor Kesteloot will contradict you adamantly: "Medicine plays a more minor role than most people are inclined to think. After all, if progress was made, how do you account for the increasing cancer mortality? People think that medical science can do a lot, whereas in reality, it fails to deliver. People don't realize the extent to which they have their health in their own hands. And this health is determined by our way of life, most importantly, by our food."

Fat consumption not only has an influence on cardiovascular mortality. Recent studies are supporting the worldwide link between fat intake and cancer. The results of a study by Professor Kesteloot on the carcinogenic effects of dairy fat are about to be published in the American journal, *Preventive Medicine*. "Had I been able to show that there is no connection whatsoever, I would also have published it," confirms Professor Kesteloot. "But there is a clear connection between the amount of saturated dairy fat consumed and the incidence of breast, colo-rectal, prostate, and even lung cancer. The best thing that could happen to us would be for cows to be banned to the zoo."

The theme of the lecture was personal and planetary health. I began by reporting on developments in America, including the National Institutes of Health study of macrobiotics and cancer. When I mentioned recent surveys showed one-third of all Americans were using alternative health care, someone stated in Belgium, *more than half* the population used alternative medicine. I also talked about *The Philosopher's Stone*, Michio Kushi's new book on alchemy and transmutation. I explained how the understanding of atomic transmutation had the potential to change science and technology and create a new industrial revolution. The first goal of this revolution is to make unlimited materials, including precious metals, available from common substances, such as air, water, and soil. The second aspect involves learning to use unlimited, non-polluting sources of energy, including the electromagnetic force, or ki, that is constantly coming in to the earth from the universe.

Paris

Early the next morning, I took a bus to the Brussels airport where I boarded the flight to Paris. I was met at the airport by Catherine and Caroline Delacoute. The Delacoute sisters have been practicing macrobiotics for over fifteen years, and are representing One Peaceful World, the international information network and friendship society started by Michio and Aveline Kushi, in France. They have studied with the Kushis and now offer macrobiotic cooking classes in Paris.

Catherine and Caroline took me on a quick tour of Paris that included a stop at a famous cafe on the Left Bank. Then we drove to the Marie Curie Institute for a meeting with a man named Professor Joyeux, one of France's top cancer specialists and a pioneer in research on cancer and diet. Professor Joyeux was in agreement with many of our ideas, especially our belief that a naturally balanced diet could help prevent many forms of cancer. Catherine and Caroline told me that he frequently appeared on French national television and recommended eating more whole grains and vegetables to prevent cancer.

Catherine, Caroline, and I boarded a train early the next morning for the south of France. Joining us was Reverend Jomyo Tanaka, a Shingon Buddhist priest from Japan who has practiced a macrobiotic way of life for many years. Reverend Tanaka lives in Vermont and is well known in the macrobiotic community. He was in France studying the parallels between Buddhism and Western religions. He was also investigating the possibility of opening a center for meditation in Paris. Reverend Tanaka was planning to lead meditation sessions every morning during my seminar in the south of France.

As the train headed south, the intensity of Paris gave way to more relaxed and expansive surroundings. South of Lyon, the gigantic cooling towers of a nuclear reactor came into view. The reactor seemed out of place with the gentle rolling hills and old-style farmhouses that dotted the countryside. Nuclear power is widely used in France. The sight of the reactor was a stark reminder of the need for creative new solutions to the environmental crisis, including increased awareness of macrobiotics.

Pezenas

We were met at the Montpellier station by Patricia Price and her daughter Rachael. Patricia and Rachael have both studied at the Kushi Institute, and, along with Catherine and Caroline, are also representing One Peaceful World in France. My friends and I stayed at Patricia's spacious home in Pezenas, a small village south of Montpellier, not far from the Mediterranean.

Patricia and Rachael took me on a tour of the area early the next morning. They explained that the southern part of France had been colonized thousands of years ago by Greek settlers. The Greeks brought olive trees to the area, and also wine grapes. The town of Pezenas is famous as the place where Moliere, the 18th century playwright and satirist, lived and produced many of his plays.

Our first lecture took place that evening in a hall in the center of Pezenas. About forty people came. Macrobiotic desserts and bancha tea were available for our guests. During the lecture, I spoke about diet and health, using the principle of yin and yang to explain how to balance our diet and lifestyle. The lecture was translated by Caroline Delacoute and Patricia Cuerot, another student of macrobiotics who had come from Paris.

A number of people came for personal consultations on the following morning. After lunch, our group—which by now included Catherine and Caroline, Reverend Tanaka, Patricia Cuerot, Patricia and Rachael, myself, and several other friends—set out for Montpellier. Patricia had arranged an afternoon lecture in Montpellier, a charming city with one of the oldest medical schools in Europe. About thirty people came to the lecture in an educational facility in the center of the city. Following the lecture we returned to Patricia's, where I lectured again that evening.

I lectured at Patricia's once more on the following afternoon. Joining us were several other macrobiotic teachers, including Jean Celle and Mateo and Helene Magarinos. Jean Celle has been involved in macrobiotic education and publishing since the Seventies. He published several of Michio Kushi's earliest books in French, including *Cancer and Diet*. He is now active in the French environmental movement. Mateo and Helene teach macrobiotics in Montpellier and throughout Europe. Mateo is well known as the translator for Michio Kushi's seminars in France.

In all, about 100 people participated in our educational programs in Pezenas and Montpellier. Patricia, Rachael, Catherine, Caroline, and I met with another cancer researcher on the following day. His name was Professor Pugols, and our meeting took place at the Val d' Aurelle Cancer Research Center in Montpellier. Professor Pugols is well known for his research on diet and cancer, and, like Professor Joyeux, we found him to be in agreement with our views on diet and cancer prevention. He was especially interested in the NIH study of macrobiotics and cancer, and stated that his work educating the public about diet and cancer would be greatly enhanced by scientific proof that a macrobiotic diet could aid in the recovery from this disease.

Alsace

Early the next morning, Patricia, Rachael, and I boarded a flight for Strasbourg in the province of Alsace. Alsace is on the border with Germany, and at various times in history has been part of France and part of Germany. Many Alsatians speak both languages and have a strong sense of independent national identity.

We were met at the airport by Michel Sheek, who, along with his wife Cecile, manages *La Miche*, a charming hotel in the mountain village of Noirceux that specializes in macrobiotic foods. Alsace was much cooler than the south of France, and there was a light cover of snow on the ground. The region is mountainous, with many chateaux and castles dotting the countryside. Alsace contains many vineyards and is internationally recognized for producing wine of exceptional quality.

    Michel explained that he started macrobiotics over fifteen years ago following a diagnosis of testicular cancer. After recovering his health, he became involved in macrobiotic education. Michel is builder by trade and did the renovations on La Miche himself. He explained that he used all natural materials in order to make the environment inside La Miche as natural, healthful, and comfortable as possible.

    I lectured that evening in the nearby town of Selestat. The lecture had been advertised in the newspaper and about 130 people came, many of whom were new to macrobiotics. The lecture had been organized by Paul Dietrich, a Catholic priest who is a teacher of macrobiotics. Paul is the head of *Terre et Partage*, the macrobiotic association in Alsace.

    Paul took Patricia, Rachael, and me sightseeing on the following morning. We went to Mount Saint Odile, a well known religious shrine dating back to the 8th century. The shrine is located on the top of a mountain, from which we were treated to a spectacular view of the mountains and villages of Alsace, as well as the Black Forest region of Germany. We all left Mount Saint Odile feeling inspired and uplifted.

    I addressed a meeting of the macrobiotic association later that day. About thirty people attended the meeting, at which Paul Dietrich served as moderator. One of our most heated discussions took place around the issue of salt. Many people in Alsace (and throughout France) are using grey sea salt. Grey salt is usually high in magnesium and this makes it too yang for daily use. It can produce an overall tightening and constricting effect in the body and mind, and lead to overly yang symptoms such as kidney stones.

    Jean-Pierre Gardette, a macrobiotic teacher from Paris who has studied in Boston, added poignant personal commentary on the importance of choosing the right salt. Jean-Pierre started macrobiotics after developing ankylosing spondylitis, a form of arthritis in which the vertebrae of the spine harden and become fused. He originally used grey salt in cooking, and this led to improvement of the more yin symptoms of his disease, especially the swelling and inflammation. However, as he continued using grey salt, his spine became tighter and it became difficult for him to walk or perform simple tasks. It was not until he came to Boston several years later and began using white sea salt that his condition slowly began to improve.

As the discussion continued, I asked Michel's wife Cecile for samples of the salt our Alsatian friends were using. She brought two samples: grey salt crystals and a somewhat refined, powdered grey salt, both from Brittany. Patricia Price had brought a bag of white salt from Baja, California (Si Salt), which is the kind we use in America. I placed each one in a bowl and asked everyone to taste all three. The difference was immediately apparent. The grey salts had a somewhat harsh, almost bitter aftertaste. The salt from Baja was mild, almost sweet, without a harsh aftertaste.

After tasting the different varieties of salt and hearing Jean-Pierre's story, many of the people in the association expressed interest in changing from grey to white salt. Patricia offered to import the Baja salt and make it available to all those in France who wanted it.

Following our discussions about sea salt, I concluded the meeting by thanking my gracious hosts and all of the members of the association. I told them that I felt inspired by the energy, vitality, and independent spirit I discovered in Alsace, and expressed my hope that Alsatian macrobiotics would become a model and a force for unity in Europe. At the end of the meeting, Michel brought out several bottles of organic Alsatian wine. He passed small wine glasses out to everyone and went around the table filling each glass. Then we raised our glasses in a rousing toast to the dream of one peaceful world.

Source: This essay is from unpublished notes and correspondence.

11.
Planetary Medicine

The macrobiotic understanding of yin and yang can help clarify the relationship between personal health and the environment. These principles enable us to see this relationship in a very dynamic and practical way, and unify our desire to heal the earth with our desire to heal ourselves. Let us see how the different parts of the environment can be classified according to the five transformations:

Energy-Stage	Environment	Organ-Pair
Upward energy (tree)	Vegetation	Liver/Gallbladder
Active energy (fire)	Solar energy: air	Heart/Small Intestine
Downward energy (soil)	Earth and soil	Spleen-Pancreas/Stomach
Condensed energy (metal)	Minerals	Lung/Large Intestine
Floating energy (water)	Oceans, lakes	Kidney/Bladder

Like the organs of the body, each part of the environment is related to the others. For example, the burning of wood and other forms of plant matter releases carbon dioxide and other substances that alter the balance of the atmosphere. Airborne pollutants eventually fall to earth, changing the quality of the soil. Pollution of the soil affects the quality of rivers, lakes, and other bodies of water, and this in turn affects trees and other forms of vegetation.

Our internal condition influences the way we relate to the different aspects of our external environment. If our condition is clear and healthy, our relationship to the environment is harmonious and self-sustaining. On the other hand, when our condition becomes stagnated and unhealthy, we begin relating to the environment in a wasteful, inefficient, and disruptive way.

For example, condition of the spleen, pancreas, and stomach influences our relationship with the soil, including our agricultural and farming practices. When these organs are sound and healthy, a person will prefer more natural methods of farming that maintain healthy, organic soil. When these organs become unbalanced, people lose confidence in natural farming and turn to pesticides and other chemicals that deplete the soil. In a similar way, the kidneys and bladder influence our relationship with water. Water pollution and the inefficient use of water resources are signs of widespread disorder in the kidneys and bladder. This relationship works both ways: foods grown in chemicalized, depleted soil weaken the spleen and pancreas, and chemically-treated or polluted water has a harmful effect on the kidneys and bladder. A similar relationship applies to the other organs and parts of the environment.

The solution to the environmental crisis lies in restoring each of the organs and the body as a whole to a normal, healthy condition. A naturally balanced, macrobiotic way of eating is the most fundamental way to restore the health of the body and ultimately correct society's mismanagement of our planetary environment. Ultimately, personal healing is equivalent to planetary healing.

Source: This essay appeared in the One Peaceful World Newsletter, *Becket, Mass., Autumn, 1994.*

12.
Toward Planetary Family

The family is our most sacred and precious institution. It predates the earliest civilizations, and has survived repeated wars, natural catastrophes, and the rise and fall of empires. It is the most durable of our social structures. Families are the cornerstone of society, the fabric out of which the web of society is woven. When families are strong and healthy, so is society. Healthy and peaceful families are the foundation of a healthy and peaceful world.

The changes in family life that have occurred during this century are a reflection of changes in lifestyle and diet during the same period, including increasing urbanization and the shift from whole to processed foods. Until 1920, the majority of Americans lived in farms, towns, and villages. By 1980, more than 80 percent were living in cities. The migration from country to city represented a more yang process in which contracting energy became stronger. The concentration of energy, activity, people, steel and concrete, and carbon dioxide in the city makes that environment more yang than the environment in the country.

The same process of contraction has occurred within the family. Before the 20th century, most people lived in extended families. In the extended family, three or four generations plus assorted relatives would live together in the same house, farm, or village. With the rise of the cities, the extended family was replaced by the nuclear family.

These two models of family life are opposite to each other. They reflect the complementarity existing between traditional rural and modern urban life. The extended family emphasized the place of individuals within the larger family unit, while in the nuclear family, individuality became paramount. The elders in the extended family taught family spirit, mutual cooperation, and the importance of working together, while in the nuclear family, the pursuit of individuality frequently disrupted harmony in the family as a whole.

Because of its rural agricultural base, the extended family was a productive unit that often achieved a surprising degree of self-sufficiency. Children were understood to contribute to the overall prosperity of the family. A large family was considered a sign of good fortune. On the other hand, the nuclear family evolved as a consumption unit lacking in self-sufficiency. From the view of modern consumers, children are thought of as liabilities, and not as blessings from nature. Today, couples often worry about how many children they can "afford," and decide to limit their number or not have any at all. Together with diet, this is a major factor in the decline of fertility among married couples.

As families moved from the country to the city, they surrendered not only their agricultural lifestyle but their traditional diet as well. Extended families nourished themselves on humanity's traditional staples: whole cereal grains, beans, fresh local vegetables, and other products of their regional agriculture. During the 20th century, families shifted from a diet based on whole grains and other complex carbohydrate foods to a diet centered around animal protein, fat, and refined carbohydrates. At the same time, naturally fertile plant and animal species were replaced by infertile, artificially fertilized, or genetically manipulated species.

These dietary changes created the underlying biological base for the decline of the extended family. While extended families ate whole, natural, and organic foods, nuclear families adopted processed, artificial, and chemicalized products. The diet of the extended family was based on locally grown, seasonal, and unrefined foods, while on the dinner tables of nuclear families, transcontinental (and recently transhemispheric), nonseasonal, and highly refined foods became predominant. The diet of the traditional, extended family centered on foods that were prepared and eaten at home, while the nuclear family relied on foods that were prepared and eaten outside the home, increasingly in fast food restaurants.

Whole grains and other complex carbohydrates provide binding power that is strong enough to hold large, multigenerational families together. More yang animal foods produce isolation that can lead to separation. A diet based on animal food leads to an unsettled, semi-nomadic existence. Extremely yin simple sugars, a major feature of the modern diet, promote fragmentation that can cause the members of a family to lose their underlying sense of unity.

Modern families have surrendered the biological high ground to the modern food industry and have lost their center; a center that for centuries was provided by home cooked meals based on whole grains and other complex carbohydrate foods.

More recently, the family has undergone increasing contraction and fragmentation. The nuclear family now makes up a minority of households in the United States. A growing number of families are headed by one parent, most often the mother. During the 1990s, about a third of all American children will be brought up by a single parent. Moreover, an increasing number of people are opting to live by themselves. During the heyday of the nuclear family in the 1950s, single person households made up fewer than ten percent of families. By 1984, the number of single person households reached 25 percent of all families in the United States, and the number has increased since then.

As we can see, the strains of modern life are causing many families to collapse. Modern eating habits have weakened reproductive ability to the point that many people are unable to produce children. As a result, couples are increasingly turning to artificial conception, including artificial insemination and in-vitro fertilization. When coupled with rising infertility rates, these techniques could lead to the appearance of totally artificial families, in which children are produced in the laboratory through reproductive technology rather than through the natural union of a man and a woman. If these techniques become widespread, the family as we know it could disappear.

Macrobiotics offers a powerful alternative to the collapse

of the family. The macrobiotic way of life embraces extended, nuclear, and single-parent families, as well as other models of family life. By emphasizing home cooking, macrobiotics can help restore a biological center to every family. A diet based on whole grains, fresh local vegetables, beans, and other complex carbohydrate foods helps secure the health of each family member. When the members of a family share healthful, home cooked meals, they begin to share the same healthy quality of blood. Sharing the same blood and spirit is what a family is all about. Macrobiotic eating can also reverse the trend toward declining fertility, by strengthening reproductive health and vitality. In traditional cultures, cereal grains are associated with fertility and abundance. That is why rice is thrown at the bride and groom at weddings.

In the natural, macrobiotic family, love and harmony are the goal of family life. This goal is symbolized by the Japanese concept of *Wa*, which we can translate as "peace" or "harmony." The character for *Wa* is made up of symbols that represent cereal grains and mouth. The ancient people who formulated this character understood that a diet based on whole grains promotes social harmony and peace. As more and more families adopt a grain-based diet, their members will come to live in harmony with each other and with the natural environment. As the number of strong and healthy families increases, we can envision a time when individuals and families throughout the world share a natural, grain-based diet, a sound and healthy quality of blood, a dream of health and peace, and a deep sense of compassion for and connectedness to the planetary family of humanity.

Source: This essay, written with Wendy Esko, appeared in Macrobiotics Today, *Oroville, Ca., March/April, 1994.*

13.
Preventing Crime through Diet

The rise of crime is one of the most pressing social concerns in modern America. Yet, of all the solutions being debated, few, if any, deal with the underlying biological causes. A look at the demographics of crime in the United States can help us gain insight into a possible cause of this modern epidemic.

People under twenty-five comprise about 40 percent of the U.S. population, yet they commit more than three-quarters of the violent crimes. People under the age of eighteen make up the majority of persons arrested for vandalism, arson, auto theft, and violation of alcohol and drug laws. Many of the burglaries and a sizable portion of the muggings in the United States are committed by young people. From 1986 to 1991, the homicide rate among 14 to 24 year olds increased by 62 percent. It rose 124 percent among those 14 to 17.

In a recent newspaper article, Scott Decker, chairman of the Criminal Justice Department at the University of Missouri, commented on the growing wave of violence among young people:

> The pattern of homicide has changed. The decreasing age of both offenders and victims is the most profound change in homicide rates since World War II.

A closer look at the statistics can shed further light on the problem. Our first observation is that the rate of violent crime is much lower among girls than boys. Secondly, there is little or no violent crime among children under ten, but around age twelve, especially for boys, the rate literally explodes upward, peaking at about age nineteen. From this peak, the rate drops rapidly. These statistics show that violent crimes are committed primarily by teenage boys. Why are teenage boys increasingly expressing themselves in such a violent and destructive manner?

During puberty, the body begins secreting sex hormones. Androgens, especially testosterone, are produced primarily in the male body, while estrogen and other female hormones are secreted in larger amounts by the female body. These hormones have a decisive influence on the physical, emotional, and behavioral changes that occur at puberty. Testosterone exerts a yang, contractive and activating effect, while estrogen exerts a yin, expansive and relaxing effect. During puberty, the male body becomes contracted and muscular, and boys begin displaying more active and aggressive behavior. Estrogen causes the female body to expand and become more well-rounded, while girls normally behave in a less aggressive manner than boys.

Among the factors influencing the secretion of these hormones, diet is of primary importance. In the macrobiotic view, production of testosterone is increased by the intake of meat, chicken, eggs, cheese and other animal foods that have a more yang or contracting effect. On the other hand, intake of milk, sugar, chocolate, and ice cream and other foods with more yin or expansive effects accelerates the production of estrogen.

In some cases, a diet high in animal foods causes the body to step up production of testosterone, and in others, it causes the body to produce stronger and more potent forms of the hormone. The high intake of animal foods, which are yang or contractive, creates disequilibrium, especially in combination with the more yang androgens secreted during puberty. The result is often an explosive discharge of yang excess, which today often takes the form of violent behavior. Although American girls also eat plenty of animal food, they produce less testosterone, and are less prone to such extreme behavior. They also discharge excess once each month during menstruation. At the same time, the hormonal surge that occurs during adolescence tends to stabilize once people reach their twenties, thus behavior becomes more stable and controlled.

The consumption of animal food has another important effect on behavior. Meat, eggs, chicken, and cheese alter the normal secretion of pancreatic hormones. The pancreas secretes two hormones: insulin (yang), which lowers blood sugar, and glucagon, or anti-insulin (yin), which cause it to rise. The excessive intake of animal food leads to blockage and stagnation in the pancreas. These strong yang foods cause the pancreas, which is a more yang, or compact organ, to become hard and tight, and reduce its secretion of anti-insulin. The result is hypoglycemia, or chronic low blood sugar.

Hypoglycemia has a direct effect on our ability to think clearly. The brain is utterly dependent upon glucose for its functioning. Low blood sugar causes the biologically less essential brain functions to shut down in order to conserve the more essential, mechanical functions. The cerebellum, which controls the more refined levels of behavior, including our sense of conscience and the ability to understand the effects of our actions, is biologically less essential than the cerebrum, which regulates breathing, heartbeat, and muscular activity of the "fight-or-flight" variety. In this condition, a person thinks less clearly and is more prone to panic or act without thought of the consequences.

Hypoglycemia caused by excessive intake of animal food also produces the craving for opposite extremes, such as sugar, alcohol, or drugs, to make balance. Alcohol abuse, fueled by hypoglycemia, is considered by many to be the leading drug problem in the United States. No less than 60 percent of the violent homicides and 40 percent of the rapes in the U.S. are alcohol related. At the same time, drug use is increasingly associated with violent crime in this country.

Writing in his book, *Diet, Crime, and Delinquency*, criminologist Alexander Shauss states that, "there is a vast medical literature suggesting the role blood sugar disorders can play in antisocial behavior." Researchers have begun to link hypoglycemia with depression, hyperactivity, and antisocial behavior. Studies of prisoners have revealed a very high incidence of hypoglycemia, as high as 85 percent in some instances, and have shown that inmates consume far more sugar and highly sugared foods and beverages than the average population.

Together with the graphic depiction and glorification of violence in the media, the easy availability of guns, and the decline of traditional family structures, the high consumption of hamburgers, fried chicken, and other forms of animal food by young people could be fueling the modern epidemic of crime and violence.

In the book *Crime and Diet* (Japan Publications, 1987), Michio Kushi and I propose a broad-based program for solving the problem of crime. One aspect involves conducting a massive dietary education program throughout the country, including lectures and cooking classes, with particular focus on high-crime areas. Dietary education could also be offered in elementary and high schools. The other aspect would be to provide dietary education in prisons, juvenile detention centers, mental institutions, and hospitals, along with reorienting the quality of food served in these institutions.

Diet has a profound influence on behavior. The value of a naturally balanced diet in the prevention of heart disease, cancer, and other chronic diseases now recognized by society. A diet of whole natural foods may also be the key to helping young people react more peacefully to the stresses of modern living, while serving as a long-term solution to the modern epidemic of crime and violence.

Source: This essay appeared in MacroChef, *Philadelphia, Pa., Late Summer, 1994.*

14.
New Reasons to be Dairy-free

In macrobiotic thinking, milk is a more yin or expansive food. Milk is a food for growth; it promotes rapid development of the newborn. Mother's milk is suitable for the earliest stages of life, but once teeth come in and a baby is able to eat grains and other vegetable foods on his own, milk is no longer necessary nor beneficial. It is at that time that the natural process known as weaning occurs, in which the young graduate to the next level of eating.

This process occurs throughout the animal kingdom. Once animals are weaned, however, they do not continue drinking milk. Man is the only species that continues taking milk beyond infancy, and the only species that takes the milk of other animals. In macrobiotic thinking, this practice is harmful both physically and spiritually.

The association between regular consumption of dairy products and a plethora of human diseases has been documented in numerous studies around the world. Now, modern science is providing consumers with additional reasons to avoid dairy foods.

Compared to animals living freely in nature, modern farm animals are often sick and weak. They live in artificial environments, under unnaturally crowded conditions, and are fed a highly synthetic diet. In order to keep these animals alive and free of infection, they are routinely fed antibiotics. Antibiotics are extremely yin; they are also given to livestock to stimulate growth. Since they are yin, antibiotics are effective against bacteria, which, among microorganisms, are more yang. They are not effective against viruses, which are more yin than bacteria. Yin and yang attract and interact with one another, whereas two yins repel and do not interact.

Just as no two people are exactly alike, no two bacteria, even within the same strain, are identical. Certain microbes within a given batch will be more yin, others more yang. The more yang varieties of bacteria will be killed by an antibiotic, whereas like viruses, the more yin varieties will not be affected. These latter bacteria, which react more like viruses, are said to be "drug resistant."

When antibiotics are applied, non-resistant bacteria are killed, while resistant bacteria survive, multiply, and even pass their resistance on to other microbes. As time goes by, an increasing number of common bacteria are evolving resistance to antibiotics. The reason for this is twofold: indiscriminate use of antibiotics by the medical profession, and the use of antibiotics in livestock. In an article entitled, "The End of Antibiotics?," *Newsweek* stated the problem as follows:

> Resistant infections killed 19,000 U.S. hospital patients (and contributed to the deaths of 58,000 more) in 1992. "Many of the diseases we thought we had under control are coming back," says the CDC's Mitchell Cohen. That's because a host of common bugs now resist one or more antibiotics. Strains of *pneumococcus*, which can cause ear infections, meningitis, pneumonia and blood infections, became resistant to penicillin and to four other antibiotics in just the last six years. Some 20 percent of TB microbes resist isoniazid, the treatment of choice, and gonorrhea microbes resist penicillin.

Regarding the role of dairy and other animal foods in the spread of drug resistant bacteria, the *Newsweek* article stated:

> Antibiotics in farm animals leave behind drug-resistant microbes in milk and meat; with every burger and shake, supermicrobes pour into your gut. There, they can trans-

fer drug-resistance to bacteria in the body, making you vulnerable to previously treatable infections.

Another new drawback to dairy food has occurred as a result of recent government approval of genetically-engineered bovine growth hormone, or recombinant BGH. Genetically-engineered growth hormone is now in use, and much of the milk, cheese, butter, yogurt, ice cream, and infant formula consumed in the U.S. will soon contain it. None of these foods will carry a label warning consumers that rBGH was used in their production.

The production of milk is a yin or expansive function. Cows injected with rBGH produce up to 20 percent more milk. Because it stimulates lactation, rBGH must therefore be extremely yin. Cows who receive rBGH are more prone to fatigue, weight loss, and mastitis, an infection of the milk-secreting udder. Researchers note up to an 80 percent incidence of mastitis in hormone-treated cows. Antibiotics are the treatment of choice for mastitis; the use of rBGH will necessitate the use of even greater amounts of antibiotics and accelerate the development of drug-resistant microbes. A Government Accounting Office report on rBGH stated: "The increase in mastitis levels reported in the rBGH pivotal studies suggests that the potential for an increase in milk antibiotic levels is very real." The use of rBGH in dairy cattle may also lead to contamination of milk with pus and bacteria.

Over the years, epidemiological studies have associated consumption of milk and other dairy products with breast cancer. The use of rBGH may increase this risk. Dr. Samuel Epstein, a noted environmental medicine specialist at the University of Illinois, stated in an article in the Los Angeles Times that rBGH increases the level of insulin-like growth factor-1, or IGF-1, in cow's milk, and that:

> IGF-1 induces rapid division and multiplication of normal human breast epithelial cells in tissue cultures. It is highly likely that IGF-1 promotes transformation of normal breast epithelium to breast cancer. IGF-1 maintains the malignancy of human breast-cancer cells, including their invasive-

ness and ability to spread to distant organs.

In nature, every action produces an opposite reaction. Every front has a back, and the bigger the front, the bigger the back. The risks associated with the use of rBGH in milk, together with the dangers resulting from a greater use of antibiotics, should cause many consumers to think more seriously about the quality of the foods they are eating and turn to more natural, vegetable-quality alternatives to dairy products.

Source: This essay appeared in The Rice Paper, Columbia, S.C., Winter, 1995.

Transmutation and Self-Sufficiency

Currently, modern nations depend entirely on the earth's natural resources as the basis for industrial society. Japan, for example, imports most of the raw materials it needs to maintain its current level of industrialization. The percentage of mineral commodities (by weight) imported by Japan in 1987 are shown in the following table:

Commodity	Percent Imported
Coal	87.66
Oil and Petrol	99.72
Natural Gas	99.94
Iron Ore	99.76
Copper	99.20
Nickel	100.00
Bauxite	100.00
Lead	91.36
Zinc	85.46
Manganese	100.00
Molybdenum	100.00
Chromium	79.39
Tungsten	82.18
Titanium	100.00

Aside from helping solve the environmental crisis, atomic transmutation could help modern nations achieve industrial self-sufficiency. If the above minerals could be produced from readily available elements, there would be no need to rely on the earth's deposited resources. Moreover, through the application of atomic transmutation, new and unlimited sources of energy may be discovered. This would free Japan and other modern nations from having to import oil, coal, and natural gas, and make each of the earth's regions energy independent.

Data on Diet and the Environment

In 1944, the last harvest before pesticides were widely used, American farmers lost 31 percent of their crop to insect and other pests. Today, after the widespread use of pesticides, according to the Iowa Green Party, Americans farmers yearly lost about 37 percent of their crop to pests. Today, 64 percent of U.S. agricultural land is used for the production of livestock feed; the grains and soybeans eaten by U.S. livestock could feed 1.3 billion people. Fifty percent of America's water resources are used for some phase of livestock production. It takes 2,500 gallons of water to produce 1 pound of meat, while only 25 gallons are needed to produce a pound of wheat. A grain-, bean-, and vegetable-based farming does not pollute the environment and is actually more efficient than chemical farming in controlling pests.

15.
Good Food and Gardening at Graterford

In the summer of 1994, I wrote an article on crime and diet, in which I updated and summarized the macrobiotic view of the connection between food and behavior, especially the effects of diet on hormones, blood sugar levels, and other factors that influence the way we think and act. The article was published in *MacroChef*, and soon afterward, I received a call from Violet Hoffman inviting me to speak on this topic at a meeting of the Organic Gardeners of Graterford, a state prison outside Philadelphia.

Violet and her husband, Jerry, are students of macrobiotics. They started the gardening club last year with the support of the prison administration, and the help of Andrea Huff, a macrobiotic friend who has done volunteer work in prisons. The Hoffmans have arranged for macrobiotic teachers to give lectures and cooking classes at the prison. The macrobiotic community has been very supportive of the project, donating time, energy, food, and books to the inmates.

On the ride to Graterford, Violet and Jerry told me there are two groups of organic gardeners at the prison. The larger, outside group is made up of men who live outside the prison walls in minimum security modular units. The smaller, inside group, is comprised of men inside the prison. Our meeting would be with the outside group. The Hoffmans mentioned that the prison was originally built to house about 2,000 inmates. Currently, Graterford is home to over 4,000 men.

The evening began with a tour of the one-acre organic garden, located just outside the prison's imposing stone walls. During the summer, the gardeners grew carrots, lettuce, squash, radishes, onions, string beans, strawberries, and watermelon according to the principles of biodynamic farming. One inmate told a local newspaper that the garden was "therapeutic" and gave him a chance to see "something you helped bring to life." The meeting was held in a small chapel right next to the prison. A gourmet natural food meal had been prepared by a Philadelphia restaurant from vegetables that were grown in the garden. Attending the dinner were about fifteen members of the gardening club along with about twenty outside supporters.

During dinner, several inmates expressed their desire to eat a more healthful diet. One inmate told a local reporter: "It's real difficult, because you have a system that doesn't promote health. Food here is cooked any old way." The menus are standardized and feature plenty of meat, sugar, and dairy food. Vegetables are cooked in butter, and meals are heated in microwave ovens. Prisoners cannot have food in their cells. In such an environment, eating well presents a formidable challenge.

I addressed the group after dinner. I began by thanking everyone for their dedication to the project. I stated my belief that the organic gardeners at Graterford were setting an example for us all. The organic gardeners are showing everyone the way to better health through natural and organic foods and relaxing outdoor activity. They are also demonstrating a practical way to restore the environment through organic farming, and showing a way for everyone to regain their spiritual connection with the earth.

We also discussed other issues, especially the difficulties the men face in trying to eat well. I expressed my opinion that access to health-supporting foods was a basic human right, like access to air, water, and sunlight, and that, like institutional food in general, the current prison diet—high in fat, sodium, and sugar—was accelerating the development of heart and other degenerative diseases. However, unlike persons in other institutions, prisoners have no other choices. They either eat what is being served, or go hungry. In a sense, by denying prisoners the right to choose health-supporting foods, society is subjecting them to a form of cruel and unusual punishment. I suggested that Graterford (and other prisons) begin providing inmates with healthful dietary choices by regularly including whole grains, beans, and fresh vegetables in its menus. Currently, the U.S. has one of the highest rates of incarceration in the world, second only to that in Russia. The number of people being sentenced to prison is increasing year by year, and overcrowding has become the rule, not the exception. Although still in its beginning stages, the Graterford project could offer America a way out of this deepening morass. Healthy people are less likely to get caught in the revolving door of crime, prison, and more crime. Instead of being breeding grounds for crime, prisons could become places of healing and self-improvement. After visiting Graterford, it became clear to me that the solution to crime will not be found in building more prisons, but in helping those in prison lead healthier and more productive lives.

Readers wishing to donate books, tapes, articles, and other study materials to the inmates at Graterford can contact Violet Hoffman, 3206 Kennedy Rd., Norristown, PA 19403-4026.

Source: This essay is from unpublished notes.

16.
Macrobiotics in the Pacific Rim

It was slightly after midnight, December 6, 1994, when my plane touched down at Singapore Changi airport. The seven-hour Tokyo-Singapore flight was the final leg of an air odyssey that started twenty-four hours earlier in Boston. Waiting for me in reception area were David Tio and Richard Seah. David, who pioneered the introduction of macrobiotics in Singapore in the early Eighties, is an alumnus of the Kushi Institute in Boston. Richard, who is vice-president of the Macrobiotic Society and publishes *The Good Life*, a colorful macrobiotic periodical, had studied in Becket. Richard had invited me to lecture in Singapore during his stay in Becket earlier in the year.

Singapore, an island-nation with a population of about three million, lies off the tip of the Malay peninsula, not far from the equator. It contains an interesting mix of ethnic Chinese, native Malaysians, and people from India. Everyone speaks English. Singapore is a fully modern metropolis with a bustling high-tech economy. Towering office buildings and high-rise apartments are juxtaposed against lush tropical vegetation.

My first teaching engagement was an evening public lecture in a large auditorium in the center of the city. The lecture was attended by about 250 people. Following the lecture, I presented a weekend workshop on Mind/Body Healing attended by about forty people, and several evening lectures, including a group consultation. In addition to people from Singapore, the seminar was attended by friends from Brunei and Bali. I saw a number of people for personal counseling, and also appeared on *AM Singapore*, a morning television show. My schedule was more or less filled from early morning until late at night.

One morning, Richard and I went to a huge food market in the "Little India" section of the city. Hundreds of stalls offered an incredible array of foods, some of which were familiar, many of which were exotic and unfamiliar. Many of the stalls sold tempeh, or whole fermented soybean cake. Tempeh is a traditional Indonesian food, and the kind sold in Singapore is available individually wrapped in the leaf used to ferment the soybeans. Unlike tempeh produced in modern sanitary facilities, traditionally made tempeh, such as that in Singapore, is covered with mold, a sign that the bacteria that synthesize vitamin B12 are active. The tempeh in Singapore was, without a doubt, the most delicious I have tasted.

Fresh tofu is also readily available, as is soymilk. Vendors sell warm soymilk as a beverage. Freshly-squeezed sugarcane juice is also commonly consumed. It is light green in color and has a dull sweet taste, very unlike the sharp, penetrating sweetness of refined sugar. It is less yin than refined sugar, and has a slight taste of chlorophyll.

Singaporeans are experiencing a variety of health problems caused by the modern diet. Singapore has one of the highest cancer rates in the world. Breast cancer, once relatively unknown among people in Asia, now affects many women in Singapore. Many Singaporeans were raised on canned, condensed milk, a remnant of British colonial days. As a result, children's sicknesses such as asthma, inner ear infections, and others are widespread. Obesity is increasingly common, including among children.

During my lectures, I referred to an article from the Physician's Committee for Responsible Medicine entitled, "Chicken is Not a Health Food." Many Singaporeans, like people in the U.S. and Europe, believe that chicken is a healthful alternative to red meat. The article points out that chicken consumption in the U.S. has increased from 14 pounds per person in 1955 to 69 pounds in 1993, largely because of the perception that chicken is more healthful than meat. In reality, however, chicken is not so different from meat. According to the article, 3.5 oz of broiled flank steak is 56 percent fat, 42 percent protein, and has 70 mg of cholesterol. Light and dark chicken with the skin contains 51 percent fat, 46 percent protein, and has 88 mg cholesterol. The most commonly eaten varieties contain between 30 percent and 60 percent fat. For optimal health, macrobiotic guidelines recommend a daily diet containing about 10 percent to 15 percent fat, mostly in the form of high-quality unsaturated vegetable oils.

Chicken is also high in protein. A serving of stewed chicken breast contains a full 75 percent protein. A high intake of animal protein contributes to osteoporosis and kidney disorders, including kidney stones, hypertension, and urinary tract infections, and is now associated with an increased risk of cancer. Researchers have known for decades that animal protein accelerates the loss of calcium from the bones. Animal protein produces an acid condition in the blood, and this activates a series of reactions that help to neutralize the acid. These reactions cause calcium to be released from the bones.

Americans eat on average 100 grams of dietary protein per day. Most studies show that more than 95 gm of protein per day results in substantial loss of calcium. This may be a primary cause of the high rate of osteoporosis in the United States and other developed countries.

Following the week in Singapore, Richard Seah, David Tio, and I made a day trip by air shuttle to Kuala Lumpur. The capital city of Malaysia is about four hours by car from Singapore up the Malay peninsula. Macrobiotic friends in K.L. had scheduled an impromptu mid-day conference for about twenty-five people at an area college. I told the group that the countries of the Pacific Rim had now arrived at a crossroads. The past twenty-five years had seen phenomenal growth in the economic and industrial development of the region. The Pacific Rim is now enjoying the fruits of material prosperity and an improved standard of living.

However, together with the new prosperity, the problems of modern civilization, including the rise of degenerative disease and destruction of the environment, are now gaining momentum. If the nations of the Pacific Rim continue to pursue technological development without self-reflection, then the negative aspects of modern civilization will only intensify. If, on the other hand, they combine technological development with an agricultural, dietary, environmental, and health revolution guided by macrobiotic principles, then the future is bright. Our friends in the Pacific Rim are in a unique position to combine enlightened dietary and environmental policy with modern high-tech development.

After a busy week in Singapore, I flew to Tokyo. I had not been to Japan since 1979, and was looking forward to my visit. While in Tokyo I stayed with Ms. Setsuko Yada and family. I had met Setsuko the summer before at the Macrobiotic Summer Conference in Vermont. She was visiting America together with about twenty-five other Japanese macrobiotic friends as a part of the annual One Peaceful World Tour.

The energy in Japan was noticeably different from that in Singapore. Japan is located in the temperate zone, Singapore, near the equator. Aside from the difference in temperature, there was a difference in environmental energy. Earth's yin, centrifugal force is stronger at the equator, due to the earth's more rapid rate of rotation there, while heaven's yang, centripetal force is stronger in the temperate zones. The strong charge of earth's force made it difficult to sleep in Singapore. It was hard to get to sleep before one in the morning, and I found myself waking up at six. In Japan, the stronger charge of downward energy, plus the cooler temperature, made me want to go to sleep by ten each night. It was also easier to sleep later in the morning.

After a day relaxing and visiting friends in Tokyo, I boarded the *Shinkansen* (bullet train) for Kyoto. I was met at the station by Mr. Junji Oba, the head of One Peaceful World Japan and the leader of the One Peaceful World Tour to America. Together we took the train to Nara. Mr. and Mrs. Oba have established a macrobiotic cooking school in Nara and arranged a lecture in a community center. About sixty people attended, mostly students of the cooking school. Mr. Oba translated the lecture into Japanese. The lecture, a general introduction to macrobiotics, seemed well-received. Following the lecture, I joined the Obas and friends for a delightful Nabe-style dinner. Mr. Oba invited me to lecture again in Nara. Like Ms. Yada in Tokyo, Mr. Oba was a kind and generous host. I returned to Tokyo the following morning and left for Boston the next day.

Macrobiotics is developing actively in the places I visited. The macrobiotic movement in the Pacific Rim reflects the dynamism of the area itself. In the future, I believe it will become easier to initiate active cooperation between the macrobiotic communities in the United States, Europe, Japan, and the Pacific Rim. During the trip, I learned many new things and gained inspiration from this unique glimpse of our emerging planetary civilization.

Source: This essay is from personal notes.

Agriculture for a Small Planet

The high maintenance efficiency of the agriculture of China, Korea, and Japan is in great measure rendered possible by the adoption of a diet so largely vegetarian. Hopkins, in his Soil Fertility and Permanent Agriculture, *makes this pointed statement of fact: "1000 bushels of grain has at least five times as much food value and will support five times as many people as will the meat or milk that can be made from it." It is clear that in the adoption of succulent forms of vegetables as human food important advantages are gained. They have a higher digestibility, thus making the elimination of the animal less difficult. Their nitrogen content is relatively higher and this in a measure compensates for loss of meat.*

—F. H. King, *Farmers of Forty Centuries* (1911)

17.
Maintaining Optimal Weight

The average person in modern society is overweight. Many people are obese. Obesity is now a problem among children as well as adults. Since the majority of modern people are overweight to one degree or another, their perception of what constitutes optimal weight is abnormal. It is well-known that thinner people live longer. People such as the Hunza in Kashmir, known for their longevity and freedom from disease, have more lean physiques. Excess weight is an acknowledged risk factor in heart disease, cancer, diabetes, and other chronic conditions. Moreover, thinner people are often more active and energetic than those who are overweight.

A broad-based macrobiotic diet provides ample calories and essential nutrients, and can help people achieve and maintain optimal weight. Foods that help in maintaining proper body weight by preventing excess weight loss include:

1. *Sweet brown rice and mochi.* Sweet brown rice and mochi (pounded sweet rice taffy) are high in protein and fat. They can be eaten often to help prevent weight loss.

2. *Fried rice or noodles.* Adding a little high-quality vegetable oil to the diet can help stabilize weight loss. Sesame oil is preferred for regular use and can be used to make delicious fried rice and noodle dishes. Tofu, tempeh, vegetables, and even fish and seafood can be added to fried rice and noodle dishes. Vegetables sauteed in sesame oil are also helpful for

this purpose.

3. *Amasake (sweet rice milk).* This refreshing beverage adds calories and fat to the diet and can be enjoyed on a regular basis. Amasake makes delicious puddings and desserts and can be used on breakfast porridges.

4. *Seitan and fu.* These wheat gluten products are high in protein and can be used regularly in macrobiotic cooking.

5. *Tofu, tempeh, and yuba.* Processed soybean products are high in protein and fat and can be eaten on a regular basis to promote optimal weight.

6. *Naturally-sweetened desserts.* Desserts such as chestnut puree, squash puddings, and cooked fruit compotes sweetened with grain sweeteners such as rice syrup or barley malt add extra calories to the diet and can enjoyed from time to time.

7. *White meat fish and seafood.* Fish is a good source of extra protein and when eaten once or twice per week helps in maintaining weight.

In addition, variety in the diet—both in terms of food selection and cooking methods—is important. A narrow diet often leads to weight loss and a decline in vitality. Too much salt or salty foods or hard, baked flour products—which cause contraction or dryness in the body—can also promote the loss of weight. It is also important to chew well, exercise on a regular basis, and prepare delicious and thoroughly enjoyable meals.

Source: This essay is from a lecture in Singapore, December, 1994.

18.
Adventures in Natural Farming

"Modern vegetables are cultivated forms of what thousands of years ago were wild grasses."
—Michio Kushi

Becket Village is approximately thirteen hundred feet above sea level. It is nestled in the Berkshire Hills, a northern branch of the Appalachian mountain range that extends from Maine to Georgia, forming the spine of America's east coast. Because of its elevation, Becket is classified as being two climate zones north of Boston, with longer winters and shorter summers. In addition to having a mountainous terrain, the Berkshires are covered with the rocky soil that New England is famous for.

It was in this environment that ten years ago, we started an organic garden on two cleared fields behind and to the side of our house. The success or failure of the garden in a particular year depended primarily on whether or not we had time to devote to tilling, planting, weeding, and generally supervising the fields. During years when our schedules were not too busy, we put more time into the garden and invariably, the results were good. In a good year, the garden provided our family with summer and winter squash, Chinese cabbage, kale, collards, carrots, radishes, cucumber, different varieties of lettuce, peas, green cabbage, broccoli, daikon, mizuna, scallions, and chives.

years ago, we decided to devote a section of the ~~tural~~, rather than organic, farming. After editing Michio's book on natural agriculture (*Healing Harvest*, One World Press, 1994), we had visions of turning all of ~~become~~ ~~village~~ into a natural garden. According to the theory of natural agriculture, as expounded in Michio's book, as well as in the writings of Masanobu Fukuoka, the famed natural farmer in Japan, once the "system" is set up, food more or less grows itself. All we have to do is go out into our fields and gardens and harvest what we need. The practice of natural agriculture is based on the philosophy of non-doing as taught by Lao Tsu. When loosely translated, "non-doing" means going along with the cycles of nature with a minimum of interference.

The first step in converting to natural agriculture is to prepare the soil. Natural agriculture is based on the concept of multicultivation. The idea is that in their original state, foods such as grains, beans, vegetables, and fruits were not isolated from natural weeds. Neatly manicured fields of wheat did not suddenly appear out of nowhere. Our food crops co-evolved with other wild plants as a part of the natural ecosystem. Isolating crops from each other and from beneficial weeds is therefore against the natural order and creates many unnecessary problems.

The benefit of having weeds co-exist with food crops is obvious. The weeds send roots into the soil that naturally soften it, eventually making tilling unnecessary. The roots hold moisture in the ground, minimizing the runoff that causes erosion. Bacteria and earthworms thrive in the root networks, making the soil rich and alive. As Michio points out in *Healing Harvest*, "healthy soil is a living thing." This type of soil can support a wide variety of food crops.

The first thing we had to do was to decide what types of weeds would be most beneficial. In his book, Michio suggests using clover, vetch, dandelion, plantain, burdock, and other hardy varieties. He offers two guidelines for selecting weeds: 1) they should be fairly short, so that we can identify the vegetables in the garden, and 2) they should be hardy and strong, so that they will establish themselves in the field and eventually replace taller weeds.

In the garden behind the house, we were faced with the problem of many tall weeds. In part, this was the result of putting hay on the field in the belief that it would serve as mulch by keeping the soil moist and preventing other weeds from growing. This turned out to be a mistake. The hay took root and started to grow. After one season, the field was covered with hay. (A good example of a problem caused by too much "doing.") Our goal would therefore be to seed the field with more useful weeds in the hope that they would establish themselves and replace the unwanted and troublesome hay.

The hay and other tall weeds in the garden are summer weeds. They reach full growth in August, and as the weather turns colder, begin to wither in the autumn. In his book, Michio advises seeding the fields with hardy winter weeds at the point when the summer weeds are beginning to fall down. As he puts it:

> If you know your land, you will know when the weeds fall down, perhaps around the middle of October. Go into your field at that time, and one or two days before you believe rain is coming, seed the land with clover mixed with the seeds of several other weeds. When rain comes, it will push the seeds down into the soil and provide them with moisture. Then, when the summer weeds fall, they provide cover and nourishment for the seeds.

The idea is that the taller weeds will not come back as strongly the following spring. If you seed beneficial weeds several years in a row, they will eventually take over the whole field and the cause the tall weeds to diminish.

During the first week of September, we sowed ten pounds of Canadian red clover (obtained from Johnny's Seeds in Maine) in both the back and side gardens. The fields were thick with summer weed growth. The back garden, where we had put the hay, was especially thick. The seeds were sown following a light rain. Additional rain fell later in the day, and a brief thunderstorm occurred on the following day. Some of the seeds were scattered over the tall summer weeds. The rain was beneficial in that it washed seeds caught on the leaves of the summer weeds down to the surface of the ground. Other seeds were sown directly on the earth. It took about one hour to scatter the clover seeds on both gardens.

Several days later, we scattered several pounds of hairy vetch and ryegrass seed (also obtained from Johnny's) on the back and side gardens. The weather was partly cloudy and the temperature in the '60s. We also picked wild burdock seeds from young wild plants growing behind our barn and scattered several small buckets of seeds on both gardens. The total time involved in this task was about two hours.

In order to establish natural agriculture on these fields, it will probably be necessary to repeat the seeding of beneficial weeds for several more years. It may take three or four years for the new weeds to establish themselves before we begin to introduce vegetables. This spring, we may introduce several varieties of beneficial spring weeds in addition to the autumn and winter seeds that were already sown. As we are discovering, natural agriculture requires patience and a long view. It is difficult to set up natural agriculture if you expect your land to begin producing right away.

This year, our plan is to continue with natural agriculture on part of the land, and to use the remaining portion for conventional organic farming. In this way we can have a supply of fresh produce during the summer, while continuing with our experimentation. As the natural agriculture portion becomes established, our hope is to transfer all of the land to this method, and to extend the natural agriculture fields to other portions of the property currently not under cultivation. Perhaps in another thirty years, the entire village of Becket will become a natural garden. It is our hope that these first tentative steps toward natural farming will inspire others to try it as well.

Source: This essay, written with Wendy Esko, appeared in Macro Chef, *Philad., Pa., Spring, 1995.*

19.
Freedom for Health

In 1994, the Massachusetts Dietetic Association sponsored legislation that would have severely restricted the right to give or receive nutritional counseling in the state. Under the proposed bills, only registered dietitians who met the standards of the American Dietetic Association (as well as physicians and nurses who were exempt) would have been allowed to give dietary or nutritional advice. In response to these attempts to restrict nutritional freedom, a coalition of nutritionists, naturopaths, homeopaths, herbalists, macrobiotic teachers and other holistic practitioners led a campaign to uphold dietary freedom of choice by convincing legislators that the bill was monopolistic and regressive.

As a result of a coordinated campaign by the American Dietetic Association, thirty-two states have approved some form of nutritional licensing. In twenty-one, mandatory laws are in effect, prohibiting or curtailing holistic practices. Below is the testimony I presented to the Massachusetts State Legislature during the April 1994 hearing on the bill.

> I speak today as a concerned citizen on behalf of thousands of people throughout the Commonwealth opposed to the bill recently put forward by the Massachusetts Dietetic Association. It is important for you, the members of the Health Care Committee, to be clear about what the dietitian licensing bill would do, since there seems to be a great deal of confusion about it, even among registered dietitians.
>
> I am not opposed to dietitians upgrading their li-

censing procedures, receiving third party reimbursement, or improving the quality of food served in hospitals, prisons, and other public institutions. I am, however, strongly opposed to dietitians attempting to monopolize the continually evolving field of nutrition. Monopoly is bad enough when it involves non-essential goods or services. It is intolerable when it comes to something as basic as freedom of choice in diet. Simply put, the dietitian-licensing bill as it now stands is regressive, monopolistic, and anti-choice. It is a clear example of a special interest attempting to override the public interest.

There is no scientific consensus as to what constitutes an optimal diet. Moreover, the public is often far ahead of dietitians when it comes to making informed nutritional choices. Thousands of people throughout the Commonwealth have lowered their intake of saturated fat, cholesterol, and refined sugar, and increased their consumption of whole grains, fresh vegetables, and other foods high in fiber without, and often in spite of, the advice of a registered dietitian. If given the choice, most citizens would choose to retain the fundamental human right to choose diet based on all the available evidence, and not only on that presented by dietitians.

I urge you, the members of the Health Care Committee, to preserve the nutritional freedoms and fundamental human rights of the citizens of Massachusetts by rejecting the dietitian licensing bill. I urge you to listen to the voice of your constituents and vote no on this restrictive legislation.

Source: This essay is based on testimony before the Health Care Committee of the Massachusetts State Legislature, April 13, 1994.

20.
Health and Spiritual Development

Designed originally according to a Buddhist mandala, or chart of the universe, the ancient city of Kyoto is considered by many to be the cultural center of Japan. It contains more shrines and temples than any other location in the country. The city is surrounded by mountains, and within its borders are many rice fields and small vegetable gardens. It escaped the bombing of World War II, and so many of its ancient structures remain. Several of the leading schools of Zen Buddhism have their centers in Kyoto, and, as Zen has continued to grow in popularity in the West, an increasing number of people from America, Europe, Australia, and other places have gone there to study.

My wife, Wendy, and I became friends with a number of these young students years ago during our stay in Kyoto, and often discussed the similarities between macrobiotics and Zen during the open house dinners that we presented in our home. One of these students, a young Englishwoman named Erica, was especially interested in the relationship between food and spirituality. Erica had gone to Japan several years earlier following a year of Yoga study in India, and at the time we met, was studying and practicing Rinzai Zen at the Dai-Toku-Ji temple in Kyoto. Although she found the practice of meditation quite fulfilling, she had nonetheless developed a number of health problems that were interfering with her practice. Her major problem had been periodic attacks of sharp pain in the middle back, for which the original diagnosis had been pancreatitis and later kidney stones. Her physician had advised surgical removal of the stones, but, at the urging of her husband, an American businessman, she decided to postpone surgery and try to heal her condition with macrobiotics.

Kidney stones, and other types of stones or cysts, develop through a simple mechanism that is dependent on how we eat and drink. The repeated intake, over an extended period, of foods such as milk, cheese, ice cream, butter, yogurt, and other dairy products, as well as meat, eggs, chicken, and refined sugar, produces a "sticky" and fat-filled bloodstream. A fat-filled bloodstream, which to some degree affects practically everyone who consumes the modern diet, could very well be the underlying cause of many illnesses, including, along with kidney stones, heart and cardiovascular disease, blood disorders, cancer, diabetes, arthritis, and others.

All of the above-mentioned foods had formed the basis of Erica's diet during childhood. However, a developing interest in Yoga led her to stop eating meat several years before she moved to Japan. She adopted a semi-vegetarian regime that had included white rice, nightshade vegetables, tropical fruits, eggs, dairy foods, and sugar. As a child, she had suffered from frequent illness, and her semi-vegetarian way of eating had not reversed that tendency. Her continuing consumption of dairy products, sugar, and eggs had produced an unbalanced condition in her body, leading to the formation of fat and mucus deposits, and these deposits formed the underlying basis for the development of kidney stones.

Kyoto is well known for having one of the hottest summers in Japan, due mostly to the tendency of the mountains that surround it to hold in heat and moisture. Following the rainy season in June, cold soda, milk, fruit juice, beer, and ice cream are consumed in great quantities. In modern Japan, where vending machines proliferate, there were many opportunities for Erica to find the additional factor required to crystallize these deposits into hard stones. The additional factor is the tendency of these fluid-like colloidal deposits to solidify when cold or iced foods or beverages are consumed.

The macrobiotic approach to kidney stones is quite simple, and, in many cases, highly successful. It involves two principal elements: (1) approaching the problem from the inside by causing the blood to clean and regenerate itself through proper diet; and (2) stimulating, from the outside, the discharge of existing stones by using simple home remedies.

When Erica first contacted me, she was in tremendous pain. It seemed that a stone had dislodged itself and gotten caught in the urinary tube. To provide temporary relief, I advised her to apply a hot ginger compress over the painful area. The heat generated by the ginger compress has the effect of activating blood circulation and producing a general expansion or relaxation of the tissues and blood vessels. The ginger compress is especially effective in cases of kidney stones, particularly to bring relief from pain that results when a stone becomes blocked in a urinary tube. The heat from the compress causes the tube to expand, thus permitting the stone to pass into the bladder. When a kidney stone becomes blocked in the urinary tube, it is advisable to dilate the blocked tube by drinking plenty of hot bancha tea or other hot liquids. In some cases, a special tea can be made by grating about a tablespoonful of fresh daikon, adding several drops of shoyu, and then filling the cup with hot water or bancha tea.

These simple remedies brought immediate relief. Within several days, Erica called for advice about her diet. I suggested that she avoid sugar, dairy food, eggs, and iced foods or beverages, and begin the standard macrobiotic diet. I advised her to continue the ginger compress and daikon-bancha tea for several days.

Erica improved steadily over the next few months, so much so that the painful spasms in her back began to disappear. As a result of her dramatic improvement, she began to introduce macrobiotics to her friends at Dai-Toku-Ji.

At one time, proper dietary practice formed an integral part of the Zen way of life, as it did with other forms of spiritual discipline. Zen monks underwent a rigorous program that including plenty of physical activity, meditation, and experiencing extremes of hot and cold weather. The cooking at

Zen monasteries was known as *Shojin-Ryori*, or "cuisine for spiritual development," and emphasized the balanced preparation of whole brown rice, fresh garden vegetables, including pickles, sea vegetables, and processed soybean foods such as miso, shoyu, and tofu. Had Erica gone to Japan a hundred years ago, there is a good possibility that she would have cured her condition as a result of living at a Zen monastery.

The purpose of this more natural way of life was to bring a person into a state of physical, mental, and spiritual health as the foundation for attaining an intuitive and spontaneous awareness of the order of the universe. The awareness of the order of the universe is referred to in Zen as *satori*. A balanced natural diet provided the foundation for achieving spiritual awareness. At the same time, Buddhist monks were traditionally noted for their robust health and longevity. In recent times, however, the tradition of Shojin-Ryori has been modified, due to the influence of modern techniques of food processing and transportation. Instead of organic brown rice, many temples in Japan serve white rice, while white sugar, once unknown in Japan, has found its way into some Shojin recipes.

Students of Zen, in particular, are well aware that it is very difficult to sit for any length of time in the cross-legged lotus position or in the seiza meditation posture if they are troubled by arthritis of if their joints are stiff and swollen. Good health is obviously necessary for activities such as these, but what is the most sure way to achieve health? Good health begins from the food choices we make each day. A balanced natural diet creates the optimal condition for the purification of our blood, cells, and consciousness. As each cell and our organism as a whole begins to function in harmony with the solar system, the galaxy, and neighboring planets and distant constellations, as well as with more immediate natural cycles of weather and planetary motion, we achieve, in addition to physical health, the realization that we are always one with the infinite order of the universe. That realization is the aim of spiritual development.

Source: This essay, from Macrobiotic Cooking for Everyone, *was published in* MacroChef, Philadelphia, Pa, Autumn, 1994.

21.
Yuki Nabé

Ingredients and Utensils:
1 1/2 cup fresh daikon radish
1/3 cup tofu, cubed
pinch of sea salt
small or medium-sized clay Nabé pot with lid
Japanese-style vegetable knife
vegetable grater (for fine grating)

Preparation:
1. Peel and finely grate daikon.
2. Place grated daikon in Nabé pot.
3. Add a small pinch of sea salt.
4. Cover and place on a medium flame.
5. Cook for 3 to 5 minutes.
6. Slice tofu into cubes.
7. Place in Nabé pot with grated dakion.
8. Cover and cook for 3 to 5 minutes.
9. Remove cover and serve.

Yuki Nabé or *Snow Nabé* can be eaten by itself, with leftovers, or as part of a meal. Yuki Nabé is delicious as is, and doesn't require additional seasoning. The above recipe serves two people.

This dish is good for softening hardened deposits of fat in the body. It helps melt away stagnation (just like melting snow), relax inner tension, and establish active energy flow. The name *Snow Nabé* comes from the almost pure white color of the dish.

Resources

One Peaceful World is an international information network and friendship society devoted to the realization of one healthy, peaceful world. Activities include educational and spiritual tours, assemblies and forums, international food aid and development, and publishing. Membership is $30/year for individuals and $50 for families and includes a subscription to the One Peaceful World Newsletter and a free book from One Peaceful World Press. For further information, contact:

>One Peaceful World
>Box 10, Becket, MA 01223
>(413) 623–2322
>Fax (413) 623–8827

The Kushi Institute offers ongoing classes and seminars including Shiatsu classes and workshops. For information, contact:

>Kushi Institute
>Box 7, Becket MA 01223
>(413) 623–5741
>Fax (413) 623–8827

Recommended Reading

1. Esko, Edward. *Notes from the Boundless Frontier* (One Peaceful World Press, 1992).
2. Esko, Edward. *The Pulse of Life* (One Peaceful World Press, 1994).
3. Esko, Wendy. *Introducing Macrobiotic Cooking* (Japan Publications, 1978).
4. Esko, Wendy. *Macrobiotic Cooking for Everyone* (with Edward Esko, Japan Publications, 1980).
5. Esko, Wendy. *Rice Is Nice* (One Peaceful World Press, 1995).
6. Kushi, Michio. *Basic Shiatsu* (with Edward Esko, One Peaceful World Press, 1995).
7. Kushi, Michio. *Forgotten Worlds* (with Edward Esko, One Peaceful World Press, 1992).
8. Kushi, Michio. *Healing Harvest* (with Edward Esko, One Peaceful World Press, 1994).
9. Kushi, Michio. *Holistic Health Through Macrobiotics* (with Edward Esko, Japan Publications, 1993)
10. Kushi, Michio. *Nine Star Ki* (with Edward Esko, One Peaceful World Press, 1991).
11. Kushi, Michio. *The Philosopher's Stone* (with Edward Esko, One Peaceful World Press), 1994.
12. Kushi, Michio. *Spiritual Journey* (with Edward Esko, One Peaceful World Press), 1994.

For a free catalog of macrobiotic books available by mail order, please write One Peaceful World Press, Box 10, Becket, MA 01223 or telephone (413) 623-2322.

About the Author

Edward Esko is one of the leading teachers and practitioners of macrobiotic philosophy and health care in the world today. He has trained extensively with Michio Kushi for over twenty years, including three years of residential study in Brookline from 1973-76. Through his activities as vice president of the East West Foundation in Boston, he played a key role in starting the natural health revolution in the 1970s, by initiating annual conferences on macrobiotics and cancer and editing publications such as *Natural Healing through Macrobiotics* (with Michio Kushi) and *Cancer and Diet*. Edward is co-founder of the Macrobiotic Summer Conference, having started and managed the Amherst Summer Program from 1975-78.

Edward has given thousands of lectures and counseling sessions over the past twenty years, and has guided thousands of people, including many with chronic illness, toward greater health and happiness. He has lectured at the United Nations in New York, in England, Scotland, France, Holland, Belgium, Germany, Czechoslovakia, Japan, Singapore, Malaysia, and Argentina, and in cities and towns throughout the United States and Canada. Edward is the co-author, with Michio Kushi, of *Holistic Health through Macrobiotics, Nine Star Ki, Basic Shiatsu, Spiritual Journey, Healing Harvest,* and other books. He is co-founder of One Peaceful World Press, the leading publisher of macrobiotic books today, and author of *Healing Planet Earth, Notes from the Boundless Frontier,* and *The Pulse of Life*.

Edward teaches regularly at the Kushi Institute's Way to Health and Dynamics of Macrobiotics programs, and recently began offering the poplular Women's Health Seminar throughout the U.S. He lives in Becket, Mass. with his wife, Wendy, also a teacher of macrobiotics, and their eight children.

Index

Acid rain, 13
Adrenaline, 25
Agriculture, 57, 81-84
Air pollution, 56-57
Alchemy, 44
Alsace, 53-55
Alternative medicine, 50
American Dietetic Association, 85
Antibiotics, 66-69
Antwerp, 49-51
Artificial insemination, 60
Atomic bomb, 47
B-vitamins, 28-29
Bacteria, 67
Becket, 81, 84
Behavior, and diet, 24-29, 63-65
Beta-carotene, 33-34
Biodiversity, 13
Biological Transmutations, 44
Bovine growth hormone, 68-69
Breast cancer, 33, 50, 68, 75
Buddha, 38-39, 78
Buddhism, 15, 51, 78, 87-90
Burkitt, Denis, 31
Calcium, loss of, 76
Campbell, T. Colin, 30-35
Cancer and Diet, 53
Cancer, 32, 33, 35, 50, 51
Chaplin, Charlie, 18
Chewing, 19, 80
Chicken is Not a Health Food, 75
Children's sicknesses, 75
China Health Study, 30-31
Circle of Seven, 46, 48
Colorectal cancer, 50
Copernicus, 22
Crime and Diet, 65
Crime,
    causes of, 65
    rise of in America, 62-63
Cyclotron, 47
Daikon-bancha tea, 89
Dairy,
    and cancer, 50, 68
    and illness, 66-69, 75
Darwin, Charles, 22
Depression, 25-27
Diet
    and behavior, 63-65
    ecological principles of, 7
Diet, Crime, and Delinquency, 64
Dietary diversity, 13
Dietary fat, 32-33
Dietitian licensing, 85-86
Drug-resistant bacteria, 67
Ecclesiastes, 37-38
Emotions, and diet, 14
Environment, 56-57
Extended family, 58-59
Factory farming, 66-68
Fever, 12
Five transformations, 56-57
Food
    as energy, 11-12
    healing power of, 19, 91
Ford, Henry, 18
Freedom of choice, 85-86
Fukuoka, Masanobu, 82
Galileo, 22
Genesis, 23, 37
Genistein, 33
Ginger compress, 12, 89
Good Life,The 74
Graterford State Prison, 71-73
Hahnemann, Samuel, 19
Healing Harvest, 81
Heraclitus, 39
Hippocrates, 30
Hoffman, Violet and Jerry, 71-73
Homeopathy, 19
Hunza, 14, 79
Hydrogen bomb, 47
Hyperactivity, 25
Hypoglycemia, 25-26, 64-65
IGF-1, 68
In-vitro fertilization, 60
Jesus, 38

Kervran, Louis, 43-46, 48
Kesteloot, Hugo, 50
Kidney stone, 12, 88-89
Kuala Lumpur, 76-77
Kushi Institute, 36, 45
Kushi, Aveline, 51
Kushi, Michio, 43, 44-45, 48, 50, 53, 65, 81-82
Kyoto, 20, 45, 87-88
Lao Tsu, 39, 82
Law of infinitesimals, 19
Logarithmic spiral, 22-23
Lung cancer, 50
Macrobiotics in prison, 71-73
Marie Curie Institute, 51
Massachusetts Dietetic Association, 85
Mastitits, 68
Matsuda, Michel, 45-46
Meditation, 15
Milk, 66-69
Mineral deficiencies, 28
Miso, 33
Mochi, 79
Modern Times, 18
Moliere, 52
Montpellier, 52-53
Nara, 77-78
Natural agriculture, 81-84
Neurotransmitters, 24
Nightshades, 10, 14
Nihon Shoki, 38
Nixon, Richard, 35
Non-doing, 82
Nuclear family, 58-60
Nuclear power, 52
Nuclear proliferation, 47
Nurses Health Study, 32
Nutritional freedom, 85-86
Oba, Junji, 77-78
Obesity, 79
Ohsawa, George, 10, 16, 35, 43-48
Oppenheimer, J. Robert, 47
Organic gardening, 71-73
Osteoporosis, 76
Other Dimensions, 45
Paris, 51-52
Penicillin, 67
Philosopher's Stone, The, 43, 45, 50
Philosopher's stone, 43
Physician's Committee, 75
Phytoestrogens, 33
Pollution, 56-57
Price, Patricia, 52-55

Prostate cancer, 50
Protease inhibitors, 33
Protein, 10, 76
Radioactive waste, 47
rBGH, 68-69
Resistant infections, 67
Salt, 54-55
Satori, 90
Schizophrenia, 27-29
Seasonal change, 8
Seitan, 80
Serotonin, 24
Sesame oil, 79
Seven Samurai, 46
Shauss, Alexander, 64
Shingon Buddhism, 51
Shojin-Ryori, 15, 89-90
Singapore, 74-77
Single parent families, 60
Soymilk, 75
Spiral, 21-23
Spirituality, 15, 87-90
Staff of life, 10
Strasbourg, 53
Sugar, 25, 28
Sugarcane, 75
Supplements, 34
Sweet brown rice, 79
Tamoxifen, 33
Tanaka, Jomyo, 51-52
Tao Teh Ching, 39
Taoism, 15
Tempeh, 75, 80
Testoserone, 63
Tofu plaster, 13
Tofu, 33, 75, 80. 91
Tomatoes, 10
Transmutation, 43-48, 69-70
Violent crime, 62-64
Virus, 67
Vitamin A, 33-34
Vitamin B12, 75
War on Cancer, 35
Water pollution, 57
Weaning, 66
Weight, management of, 79-80
Whole foods, 34-35
Women's Health Trial, 32
Yin and yang, 11, 21, 26, 38, 41-42, 56-57, 63-64, 66-68
Yuba, 80
Yuki Nabe, 91
Zen, 87-90

Basics & Benefits of Macrobiotics

Essays on the Macrobiotic Way of Personal and Planetary Health

By Edward Esko
Foreword by Alex Jack

One Peaceful World Press
Becket, Massachusetts

Basics & Benefits of Macrobiotics
© 1995 by Edward Esko

All rights reserved. Printed in the United States of America. No part of this book may be used or reproduced in any manner whatsoever without written permission except in the case of brief quotations embodied in critical articles or reviews. For information, contact the publisher.

For further information on mail-order sales, wholesale or retail discounts, distribution, translations, and foreign rights, please contact the publisher:

One Peaceful World Press
P.O. Box 10
Leland Road
Becket, MA 01223
U.S.A.

Telephone (413) 623-2322
Fax (413) 623-8827

First Edition: September 1995
10 9 8 7 6 5 4 3 2 1

ISBN 1-882984-14-5
Printed in U.S.A.